CHIEVE YOUR DREAM BODY

HE ULTIMATE QUIDE TO ACHIEVING THE PERFECT BODY AND CHANGING YOUR 'EALTH LIFE STYLE IN 90 DAYS

his is the most comprehensive guide ever, with everything I have learned in 10+ ears dedicated to helping you reach your health and fitness goals.

rom everything you need to know and understand before starting your starting our fitness journey, including tips for weight loss, muscle growth, peach perfect utt, proper nutrition as well as healthy food swaps.

ll detailed to include specific exercises targeting specific muscles, programs to ɔllow depending on your fitness needs as well as types and examples of food to ubstitute for unhealthy cravings.

/HAT TO EXPECT

- Save time researching the many unclear articles on the Internet about what really works.
- Confidence that you are making the right decision with your fitness goals.
- Easy to follow programs even on a tight schedule.
- Proper scientifically proven food nutrition
- Loose weight or gain muscle without having to count calories
- Easy and fun to follow workouts for any environment and any level of fitness
- Workout without fear of injury or improper form
- How to listen to your body and follow what really work for you: Remember what works for others might not be what works for you.
- No more going hungry or spinning your wheels in the gym
- Reach your fitness goals while enjoying your life.

ABOUT THE AUTHOR

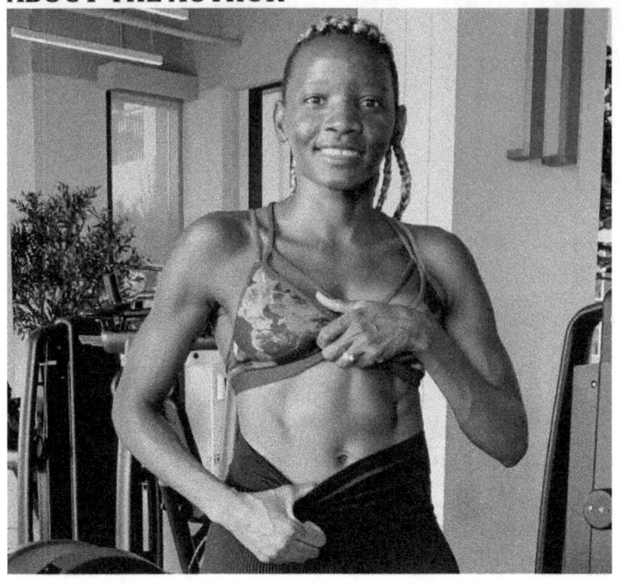

Hey, I am Hambeleleni, and just like you I have spend years confused about health, fitness and nutrition.

Growing up in a small village in Namibia, I have always been a sports lover. I started at a really young age, competing at school in running both long and short distance. In general I played most of the sports that where available to me including, volleyball, basketball, netball, high jumps, long jumps as well as soccer.

After completing high school and moved to university in the city, I got a chance to register for a local gym, but since I didn't have much money to pay for a personal trainer, I decided to learn everything by my self, which let me tell you, was not as easy as I though. All of the information on the Internet is not very well informative.

My goal from the very start was to gain some muscles and tone my body, as I have always been very skinny regardless of what or how much I ate.

After completing university I got offered a job to move all the way to Dubai. It was like a dream come true. My first few years in Dubai I turned into a party freak, partying every day of the week and neglecting my health and paying for it.

Once I started prioritizing my health, everything has changed. It took me years of trail and error. I wish I had someone to teach me what I am about to share with you in this e-book.

I have spend years researching, studying and practicing what I am finally sharing with you in this guide.

TABLE OF CONTENT

1. INTODUCTION

Walking, lifting weights, doing chores- it's all-good. Regardless of what you do, regular exercise and physical activities is the path to health and well-being. Exercise burns fat, build muscles, lowers cholesterol, eases stress and anxiety, and lets us sleep restfully. In this guide, I match all resources to help you understand and get started with your fitness journey, at every fitness level.

WHAT IS FITNESS

Fitness is defined as the quality or state of being fit. Modern definition of fitness describes either a person or machine's ability to perform a specific function or a holistic definition of a human's adaptability to cope with various situations. This has led to an interrelation of human fitness and attractiveness, which has mobilized the global fitness and fitness equipment industries. Regarding specific functions, fitness is attributed to personnel who possess significant aerobic and anaerobic ability, i.e. strength and endurance.

A holistic definition is define by Greg Glassman in the Cross fit journal as an increased work capacity across board times and modal domains; mastery of several attributes of fitness including strength, endurance, power, speed, balance and coordination and being able to improve the amount of work done in a given time with any of these domains. A well-rounded fitness program will improve a person in all aspects of a person, rather than one such as on cardio, respiratory endurance or only weight training.

A comprehensive fitness program tailored to an individual typically focuses on one or more specific skills and on age, or health related needs such as bone health. Many sources also cite mental, social and emotional health as an important part of overall fitness.

This is often presented in textbooks as a triangle made up of three points, which represent physical, emotional and mental fitness. Physical fitness can also prevent or treat many chronic health conditions brought on by unhealthy lifestyle or aging. Working out can also help some people sleep better and possibly alleviate some mood disorders in certain individuals.

Developing research has demonstrated that many of the benefits of exercise are mediated through the role of skeletal muscle as an endocrine organ. That is, contracting muscles release multiple substances known as myokines, which promote the growth of new tissue, tissue repairs, and various anti-inflammatory functions, which in turn reduce the risk of developing various inflammatory diseases.

2. FITNESS PRINCIPLES

A) Strength Training

If you knew that a certain type of exercise could benefit your heart, improve balance, strengthen bones and muscles, and help you lose or maintain weight, wouldn't you want to get started? Well, studies show how strength training can provide all those benefits and more.

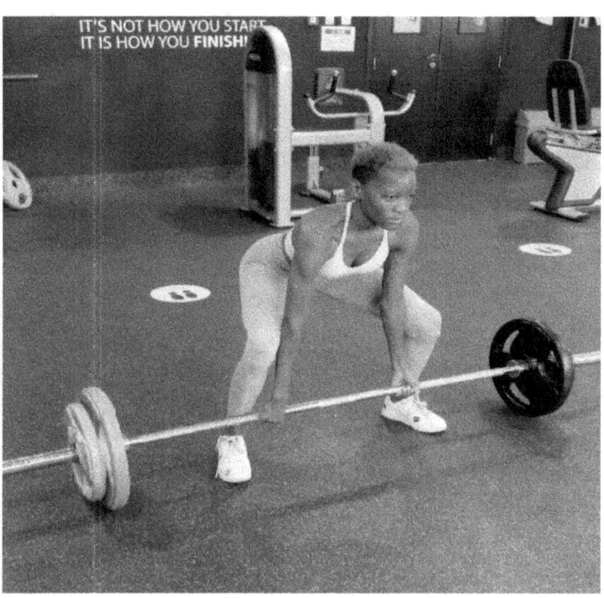

Strength training- also known as a weight or resistance training- Is physical activities designed to I prove muscular strength and fitness by exercising a specific muscle or muscle group against external resistance, including free-weights, weight machines, or your own body weight, according to the American Heart Association.

The basic principle is to apply a load and overload the muscle so it needs to adapt and get stronger. And what's important for everyone is that strength training is not just about builders lifting weights in a gym. Regular strength training or resistance training is good for people of all ages and fitness level to help prevent the natural loss of lean muscles mass that comes with aging (the medical term for this is sarcopenia). It can also benefit people with chronic health conditions, like obesity, arthritis or a heart condition.

For some people, the phrase strength training is intimidating, but it's enhancing your ability to move safely and effectively in your life. For example... the ability to lift something and put it on shelf, carry your groceries in the door, bend down and pick up something or get up after you have fallen down. Getting up off the floor requires you to recruit muscles in your upper body, abs, legs and gluteus.

You don't get better during workouts you get better in between. You should give yourself a day in between strength training to allow your body to recover and rebuild the muscle tissue from the stimulus of lifting or resistance.

How Strength Training Helps Your Health

Besides the well-touted (and frequently instagrammed) benefit of adding tone and definition to your muscles, how does strength training help? Here are just a few of the many ways:

1. **Strength Training Makes You Stronger and Fitter**

This benefit is the obvious one, but it shouldn't be overlooked. Muscle strength is crucial in making it easier to do the things you need to do on a day-to-day basis, especially as we get older and naturally start to lose muscles.

Muscle strength is also called resistance training because it involves strengthening and toning your muscles by contracting them against a resisting force. According to the encyclopedia of Behavioral Medicine, there are two types of resistance training:

- ***Isometric resistance-*** Involves contracting your muscles against a non-moving object, such as against the floor in a push up.
- ***Isotonic resistance training-*** Involves contracting your muscles through a range of motion, as in weight lifting.

2. **Strength Training Protects Bone Health and Muscle Mass**

At around age 30 we start losing as much as 3 to 5% of lean muscle mass per decade due to aging. According to a study published in October 2017 in the Journal Bone and Mineral Research, just over 30 minutes twice a week of high intensity resistance and impact training was shown to improve functional performance, as well as bone density, structure and strength in postmenopausal women with low bone mass, and it had no negative effects.

Likewise, the HHS physical activity guideline note that, for everyone, muscle strengthening activities help preserve or increase muscle mass, strength, and power which are essential for bone, joint and muscle health as we age.

3. **Strength Training Helps Your Body Burn Calories Efficiently**

All exercises help boost your metabolism (the rate your resting body burns calories throughout the day). With both aerobic activity and strength training, your body continues to burn calories after strength training as it returns to its more restful state (in terms of energy exerted).

But when you do strength, weight, or resistance training, your body demands more energy based on how much energy you are exerting (meaning the harder you are working out, the more energy is demanded). So you can amplify this effect depending on the amount of energy you put into the workout. That means more calories burned during the workout, and more calories burned after the workout too, while your body is recovering to a resting state.

4. **Strength Training Helps Keep the Weight off for Good**

Because strength training boost excess post-exercise oxygen consumption, it can also help boost weight loss more than if you were to just do aerobic exercise alone. Resistance or strength training keeps your metabolism active after exercise, much longer than after an aerobic workout.

That is because lean tissue in general is more active tissue. If you have more muscle mass, you will burn more calories- even in your sleep, that if you didn't have that extra lean body mass. A study published in found that, compared with dieters who didn't exercise and those who did only aerobic exercise, dieters who did strength training four times a week for 18 months lost the most fat.

You may even be able to further reduce body far specifically when strength training is combined with reducing calories through diet. People who followed a full body resistance training and diet over the course of up to 4 months reduced their fat mass while improving lean muscle mass better than either resistance training or dieting alone.

5. **Strength Training Helps You Develop Better Body Mechanics**

Strength training also benefits your balance, coordination, and posture. According to a review in Aging Clinical and Experimental Research in November 2017, doing at least resistance training session per week, performed alone or in a program with multiple different types of workouts, produced up to a 37% increase in muscle strength, a 7.5% increase in muscle mass and a 58% increase in functional capacity linked to risk of falls in frail, elderly adults.

Balance is dependent on the strength of the muscles that keep you on your feet. The stronger those muscle, the better the balance.

6. **Strength Training Can Help With Chronic Disease Management**

Studies had shown that strength training could also help ease symptoms in people with many chronic conditions, including neuromuscular disorders, chronic obstructive pulmonary disease and some cancer among others.

For people suffering from diseases such as type 2 diabetes, strength training along with other healthy lifestyle changes can help improve glucose control, according to the Center for Diseases Control and Prevention and a study published in June 2017 in Diabetes Therapy.

7. **Strength Training Boosts Energy Levels and Improves Your Mood**

Strength training has been known to be a legitimate treatment option or an add-on treatment to cure symptoms of depression, according to an analysis of 33 clinical trials published in JAMA Psychiatry in June 2018.

All exercise boosts mood because it increases endorphins. But for strength training according to several studies, such workouts have a positive effect on the brain. And there is evidence that strength training may help you sleep better. And we all know a better night's sleep can go a long way in keeping the mood up.

8. Strength Training Has Cardiovascular Health Benefits

Along with good aerobic exercise, muscle-strengthening activities helps improve blood pressure and reduce risk of hypertension and heart disease according to HHS.

B) Endurance training

Endurance training is one of the four types of exercise along with strength, balance and flexibility. Ideally all four types of exercise would be included in a healthy workout routine.

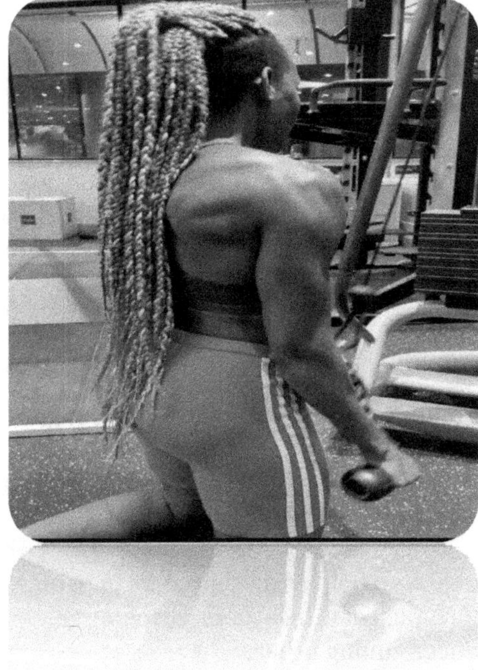

They don't need to be done everyday, but variety helps keep the body fit and healthy, and makes exercise interesting. You can do a variety of exercises to keep the body fit and healthy and to keep your physical activity routine exciting. Many different types can improve your balance, strength, endurance and flexibility. For example practicing yoga can improve your balance, strength and flexibility. A lot of lower-body strength-training exercises also will improve your balance.

Also called aerobic exercise, endurance exercise includes activities that increase your breathing and heart rate such as walking, jogging, swimming, biking and jumping rope.

Endurance activities keep your heart, lungs and circulatory system healthy and improve your overall fitness. As a result, people who get the recommended regular physical activity can reduce the risk of many diseases such as a diabetes, heart disease and stroke.

How Much Do I Need?

Building your endurance makes it easier to carry out many of your everyday activities. If you are just starting out on an exercise routine after being sedentary, don't rush it. If you haven't been active for a long time, it's important to work your way up over time.

Start out with 10-15 minutes at a time and then gradually build up. The AHA recommends that adults get at least 150 minutes of moderate to vigorous activity per week. Thirty minutes a day five days a week is an easy goal to remember. Some people will be able to do more. It is important to set realistic goals based on your own health and abilities.

Making Progress

When you are ready to do more, you can build on your routine by adding new physical, increasing the distance, time or difficulty or your favorite activity, or do your activities more often. You could first build up the amount of time you spend doing endurance activities, then build up the difficulty of your activities. For example, gradually increase your time to 30 minutes over several days to weeks by walking longer distance. Then walk more briskly or up hills.

Example of endurance exercise:

- Walking briskly
- Running or jogging
- Dancing
- Biking
- Climbing stairs at work or at home

C) Balance Training

Though it might not cross your mind, you need good balance to od just about everything, including walking, getting out a chair and leaning over to tie your shoes. Strong muscles and being able to keep yourself steady make all the difference in those and many other things you do everyday.

IT'S NOT HOW YOU START...
IT IS HOW YOU FINISH!

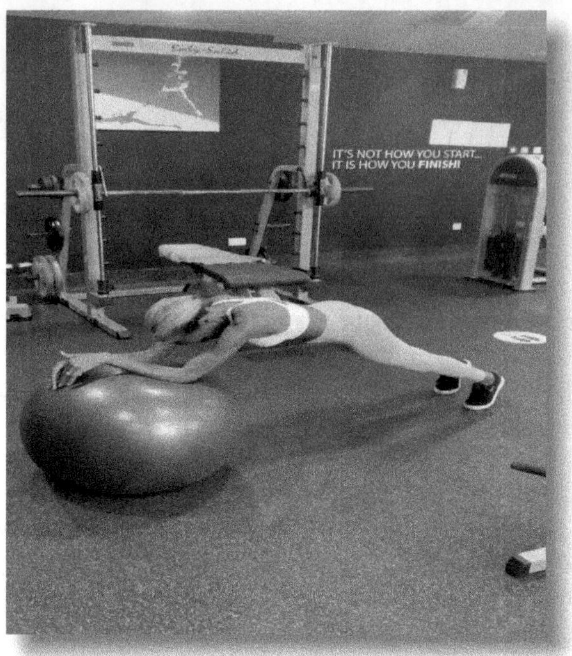

Balance training involves doing exercises that strengthen the muscles that help keep you upright, including your legs and core. These kinds of exercises can improve stability and help prevent falls.

Doing balance exercise can be intense, like some very challenging yoga poses. Others are simple as standing on one leg for a few seconds. Or you can use equipment that forces your body to stabilize itself, like a Bosu half-circle stability ball or a balance board you use along with a video game.

Example of balance exercises includes;

- Standing with your weight on one leg and raising the other leg to the side or behind you
- Putting your heel right in front of your toe, like walking a tightrope
- Standing up and sitting down from a chair without using your hands
- Walking while alternating knee lifts with each step
- Doing tai chi or yoga
- Using equipment, like a Bosu, which has an inflatable dome on top of a circular platform, which challenges your balance

Over time, you can improve your balance with these exercises by:

- Holding the position for a longer amount of time
- Adding movement to a pose
- Closing your eyes
- Letting go of your chair or other support

You can do balance exercises as often as you'd like, even every day. Add in two days a week of strength training, which also helps improve your balance by working the muscles that keep you stable.

Intensity Level: Moderate

To balance train, you don't have to run, jump, or do any other high-impact or high-intensity exercises. Usually balance training involves slow, methodical movements.

Areas It Targets

Core: Yes. You need strong core muscles for good balance. Many stability exercises will work your abs and other core muscles.

Arms: No. Most balance exercises are about balancing on your feet. So unless you're doing moves that involve your arms, or you're holding weights, they don't work your arms.

Legs: Yes. Exercises in which you balance on one leg and then squat or bend forward also work the leg muscles.

Glutes: Yes. The balance exercises that work the legs also tone the glutes.

Back: Yes. Your core muscles include some of your back muscles.

D) Flexibility Training

Flexibility refers to the total range of motion of a joint or group of joints. Flexibility, which differs from person to person and from joint to joint, encompasses all the components of the musculoskeletal system as well as specific neuromuscular pathways of the body. The structural characteristic of the joints and the mechanical properties of the connective tissues of the muscle tendon structure largely affect the extent of movement around a given joint.

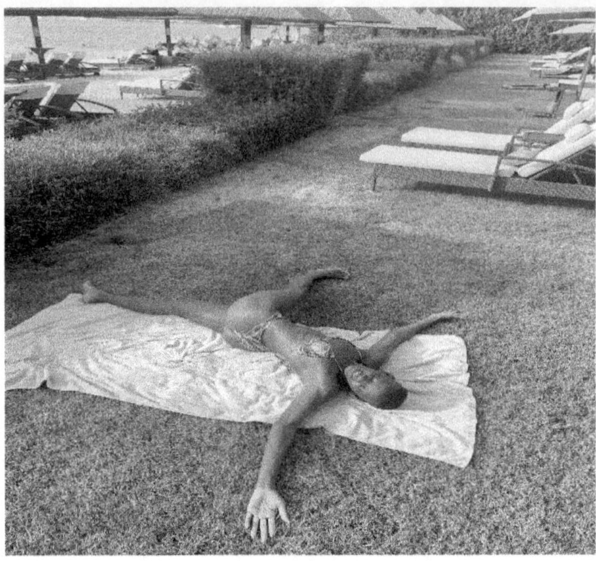

The specificity of movement that a person preforms in regular physical activities and stretching methods often define the development and improve of the body's range of motion. The goal of all stretching programs is to optimize joint mobility while maintaining joint stability. Concern should always be focused on systematic, safe and effective application of the range of motion techniques utilized.

Benefits of stretching

Studies done on flexibility found some of the following to be the befits of regular stretching:

- An increase in functional range of motion.
- Reduced low back pain and injury
- Reduction in the incidence and severity of injury
- Improvement in posture and muscle symmetry
- Delay in the onset of muscle fatigue
- Prevention and alleviation of muscle soreness after exercise
- Increase in the level of certain skills muscular efficiency
- Promotion of mental relaxation
- An opportunity for spiritual growth and self evaluation
- Personal enjoyment and gratification.

Flexibility training has more recently been recognized amongst the other components of fitness as a means to better unify one's mind, body and spirit. Taking a similar approach to the harmony of the mind, body and sprit in yoga techniques, many health practitioners are using flexibility training as a vehicle to facilitate mental and physical relaxations well as stress reduction.

Joint consideration with flexibility

The points in your body where two or more bones meet are called joints or articulations. There are three types of joints:

1. Synarthrodial joints-Allows no movement (such as in the skull)
2. Amphiarthrodial joints- Allow limited movement (such as in the spine)
3. Diarthrodial joint- Allow considerable movement (such as in the arms and legs)

The diarthrodial joints are the greatest concern in flexibility training. The diarthrodial or synovial joint (as it is sometimes called) function is to hold securely together while considerable permitting considerable movement. The adjacent ends of the bones are covered with weight-bearing or articular surface known as the articular cartilage. This cartilage absorbs shock and prevents direct wear on the bone. The composition characteristics of the articular cartilage are something between solid and a liquid.

The ligamentous sleeve called the capsular ligament is attached firmly to both bones of the joint, enclosing the joint entirely. The capsular ligament is lined with a thin synovial membrane, which secretes a synovial fluid into the joint cavity. This synovial fluid provides nourishment to the articular cartilage and serves as a lubricant to the joint. It also converts the compression stress placed upon the joint from physical activities to a hydrostatic stress, which limits the potential dangers to the joint.

In addition to the capsular ligament, each joint typically has several other ligaments that serve to help bond the bones together. The ligaments are strong fibrous bands that are made from the same tissue found in the joint capsule. Besides helping to bind the bones, ligaments serve to prevent dislocation, and limit some ranges of movement.

3. Goal Setting

Have you decided that its time to make change but aren't sure how to get started? Or have you already set more goals for yourself than you care to admit but keep failing to reach them?

No matter how big or small your goal is, whether it's losing 5 or 50 pounds, walking a mile or running your first marathon, making change requires planning and SMART goals.

Follow these guidelines to setting SMART goals and you will be surprised at what you can do:

SMART Goals:

1. Specific
2. Measurable
3. Achievable
4. Realistic
5. Timely

Some studies have shown that working towards specific, measurable, achievable, relevant and timely goals can improve your chances of achieving success.

Specific- Clearly define your goal

Effective goal setting involves more than just writing down an idea of what you want to achieve. You need to be specific. When you have a specific goal, it is easier to know if you have reached it, and to plan out the steps you need to achieve it.

For example, saying " I want to get healthy" is not specific enough. What do you define as healthy? How will you be able to tell when you are healthy? This phrase does not provide you a clear direction.

An example of a specific goal can be: I want to lose weight. Striving for this particular goal means you are working towards getting fitter and stronger. It also provides a focus for your training, which makes it easier to work towards.

Measurable: Make your goals measurable

When you can track a goal against a benchmark, you know if you are getting close to achieving your goals or not. This can motivate you to work towards a goal.

An example of a measurable goal setting could be " I want to lose 5 pounds". This gives you a specific number to measure, track and evaluate your progress toward your fitness goals and know when you have achieved it.

By specifying how many pounds you want to lose, you can measure your progress by keeping track of how much weight you have successfully lost over time.

Achievable: Goals needs to be achievable

All goals should be challenging, however, it is so important that they are also achievable. For example, setting a goal of 5 pounds in 2 weeks is probably not an achievable goal when you are just beginning.

This doesn't mean that you should no go ahead and set yourself some big goals. However you need to break those big goals into smaller, achievable goals that lead to a bigger goal.

So let's consider the goal of losing 5 pounds. If you are a fitness beginner, an achievable version might be to aim for 3 to 6 moths. You can then work towards this by setting smaller goals such as losing 2 pounds in one month, before taking new, more challenging steps to achieve the overall goal.

Relevant: Set goals relevant to you

You need to set goals that you can realistically do the work to achieve, considering your lifestyle, resources, current fitness level and available time. The goals you se should be relevant to your to your life, and appropriate for your health and lifestyle. Think about why you set the goal and why you want to achieve it in the first place. Will it improve your quality of life? Perhaps you want to feel stronger and healthier so that you can be more active: this is a meaningful goal and as a result you might be more committed to working toward it.

Similarly, if you decide to commit to five evening workouts at the gym per week when it doesn't suit your lifestyle, then this might not be a relevant or realistic goal for you. Be sure to set your goals high but make sure they suit your lifestyle.

Time-specific: Goals should be time specific

Setting a start time and a deadline for your goal is important. This allows you to work out a plan to achieve the goal by breaking it into daily actions and smaller milestones. An example of this would be to say;“ I want to lose 5 pounds by (insert date)”.

When you set yourself a realistic time frame, its easier to plan and schedule the time you'll need to dedicate towards achieving your goal, and you are more likely to be motivated to work towards a specific deadline.

Regularly reassess your progress

With any goal, it is important to keep track of your progress. You may need to be flexible- it's possible you will have to revise your ambitions if you encounter a fitness setback, or you'll have to challenge yourself if you reach goal sooner.

Find a way to track your fitness so that you can see your progress, and maintain motivation as you keep working towards your goal. If you like to have regular rewards and reminders, try using a fitness tracker to record workouts and set your daily movement goals.

Another easy way to keep track of your progress over time is to keep a journal to record whether you have achieved the smaller goals and actions that are part of your plan to achieve your bigger goals.

Now that you know how to set your SMART goals, its time to take action.

As you plan your goals, write down your reasons for selecting that goal and the specific details of the goal itself. Once you know exactly what your new fitness goal is, you can make time for exercise and map out a plan to achieve it.

When setting your SMART fitness goals, it is so important that they are YOUR goals and are meaningful and relevant to you. Don't compare your goals to others, as everyone is on an individual journey with unique challenges.

4. Guide to getting started

Starting a fitness program maybe one of the best things you can do for your health. Physical activities can reduce your risk of chronic diseases; improve your balance and coordination, help you loose weight and improve your sleeping habits and self esteem. The following steps will help you in starting your fitness program:

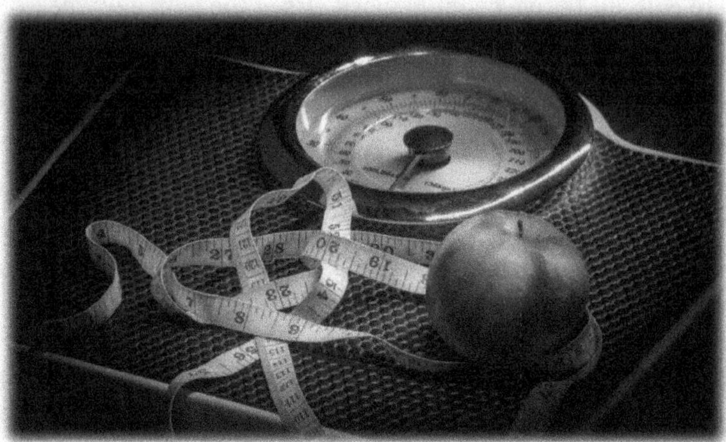

1. ***Assess your fitness level***

You probably have some idea of how fit you are. But assessing and recording baseline fitness scores can give you a benchmark against which to measure your progress. To assess your aerobic and muscular fitness, flexibility and body composition, consider recording the following:

- Your pulse rate before and immediately after walking 1 mile (1.6 kilometers)
- How long it takes to walk 1 mile, or how long it takes to run 1.5 miles (2.41 kilometers)
- How many standard or modified pushups you can do at a time
- How far you can reach forward while seated on the floor with your legs in front of you
- Your waist circumference, just above your hipbones
- Your body mass index (BMI)

2. ***Design your fitness program***

It is easy to say that you will exercise everyday. But you'll need a plan. As you design your fitness program, keep the following in mind:

- ***Consider your fitness goals.*** Are you starting a fitness program to help lose weight? Or do you have another motivation, such as preparing for a marathon? Having clear goals can help you gauge your progress and stay motivated.
- ***Create a balance routine*:** Get at least 150 minutes of moderate aerobic activities a week, or 75 minutes of vigorous aerobic activities a week, or a combination of moderate and vigorous activities. The guidelines suggest that you spread out this exercise during the course of a week. To provide even greater health benefits and to assist with weight loss or maintain weight loss, at least 300 minutes a week is recommended.

But even small amounts of physical activities are helpful. Being active for short periods of time throughout the day can add up to provide health benefits.

Do strength training for all major muscles groups at least two times a week. Aim to do single set of each exercise, using a weight or resistance level heavy enough to tire your muscles after about 12 to 15 repetitions.

- ***Start low and progress slowly.*** If you're just beginning to exercise, start cautiously and progress slowly. If you have an injury or a medical condition, consult your doctor or an exercise therapist for help designing a fitness program that gradually improves your range of motion, strength and endurance.
- ***Build activity into your daily routine.*** Finding time to exercise can be a challenge. To make it easier, schedule time to exercise as you would any other appointment. Plan to watch your favorite show while walking on the treadmill, read while riding a stationary bike, or take a break to go on a walk at work.
- ***Plan to include different activities.*** Different activities (cross-training) can keep exercise boredom at bay. Cross training using low-impact forms of activity, such as biking or water exercise, also reduces your chances of injuring or overusing one specific muscle or joint. Plan to alternate among activities that emphasize different parts of your body, such as walking, swimming and strength training.
- ***Try high-interval intensity training.*** In high-interval intensity training, you perform short bursts of high-intensity activity separated by recovery periods of low-intensity activity.
- ***Allow time for recovery.*** Many people start exercising with frenzied zeal — working out too long or too intensely — and give up when their muscles and joints become sore or injured. Plan time between sessions for your body to rest and recover.
- ***Put it on paper.*** A written plan may encourage you to stay on track.

3. Assemble your equipment

You will probably start with athletic shoes. Be sure to pick shoes designated for the activity you have in mind. E.g. Running shoes are lighter in weight compared to cross training shoes, which are more supportive.

If you are planning to invest in exercise equipment, choose something that is practical, enjoyable ad easy to use. You may want to try out certain types of equipment at a fitness center before investing in your own equipment.

You might consider using fitness apps for smart devices or other activity tracking devices, such as once that can track your distance, track calories burned or monitor your heart rate.

4. Get started

Now you are ready for action. As you begin your fitness program, keep these tips in mind:

- ***Start slowly and build up gradually.*** Give yourself plenty of time to warm up and cool down with easy walking or gentle stretching. Then speed up to a pace you can continue for five to 10 minutes without getting overly tired. As your stamina improves, gradually increase the amount of time you exercise. Work your way up to 30 to 60 minutes of exercise most days of the week.
- ***Break things up if you have to.*** You don't have to do all your exercise at one time, so you can weave in activity throughout your day. Shorter but more-frequent sessions have aerobic benefits, too. Exercising in short sessions a few times a day may fit into your schedule better than a single 30-minute session. Any amount of activity is better than none at all.
- ***Be creative.*** Maybe your workout routine includes various activities, such as walking, bicycling or rowing. But don't stop there. Take a weekend hike with your family or spend an evening ballroom dancing. Find activities you enjoy to add to your fitness routine.
- ***Listen to your body.*** If you feel pain, shortness of breath, dizziness or nausea, take a break. You may be pushing yourself too hard.
- ***Be flexible.*** If you're not feeling good, give yourself permission to take a day or two off.

5. Monitor your progress

Retake your personal fitness assessment six weeks after you start your program and then again every few month. You may notice that you need to increase the amount of time you exercise in order to continue improving. Or you may be pleasantly surprised to find that you are exercising just the right amount to meet your fitness goals.

If you lose motivation, set new goals or try a new activity. Exercising with a friend or taking a class at a fitness center may help, too.

Starting an exercise program is an important decision. But it doesn't have to be an overwhelming one. By planning carefully and pacing yourself, you can establish a healthy habit that lasts a lifetime.

5. Fitness Programs:

A) Weight loss

If you are trying to lose weight, a weight loss workout plan can be very helpful. Getting regular exercise can help you meet your goals in a healthy, sustainable way. But sometimes knowing where to start can be a very tricky situation. From how often you sweat to types of workouts you do, there are endless possibilities when you are getting into a fitness routine, and it can be a lot to think about.

Before we really get into it, we want to make it clear that weight loss as a goal isn't necessarily for everyone. For anyone who has a history of disorder eating, even if you are in recovery, you should consult your doctor before you pursue any weight ɔss goal, including starting a new exercise routine. And even if you don't have a istory of disordered eating, it's really important to have realistic expectations and ıake sure you're pursuing weight loss in a healthy way. Results can be incredibly ifficult to come by, may take a very long time to achieve and are also really hard ɔ maintain. Plus, exercise is only part of the equation. Your eating habits matter more on that below), and getting sufficient sleep and keeping many factors at lay, its no wonder weight loss is a very unique experience for every person.

Vhen it comes to the exercise part, I am here to take some of the guesswork out of ıe equation. In this chapter, I will include a weight loss workout plan. It ıcorporates the strength training, cardio and rest days you will need to reach your tness goals.

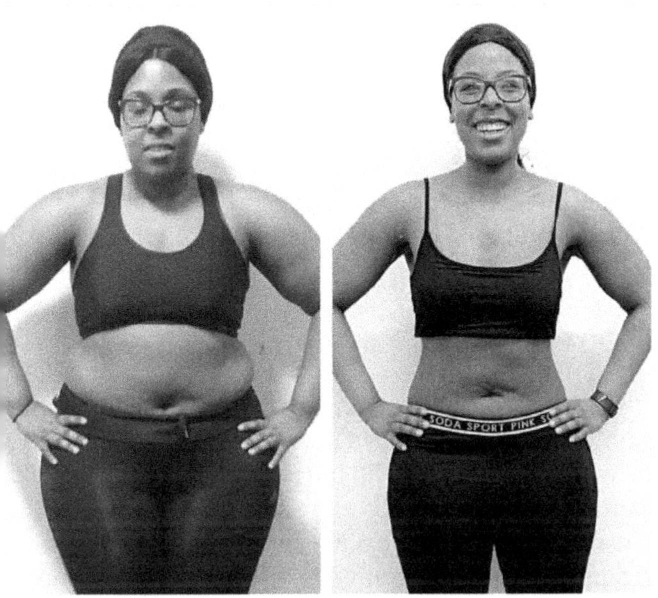

t's not enough to get out there and get sweaty: Weight loss requires strategy

can't talk about working out for weight loss without mentioning one other crucial lement of meeting your goals: Your eating habits. To create a caloric deficit that əads to weight loss, you have to eat fewer calories that you are burning. You also eed to be cognizant about what you are eating, making sure to eat quality calories nd watch portion sizes.

lutrition is priority number one- You can't out train a bad diet, 80% nutrition plus 0% training equals 100% results. (More on nutrition below) There is no need to ompletely overhaul your life at once if it feels too overwhelming at first, that's ool- just start working out and make some tweaks. Start small.

nd when it comes to working out, variety is winning factor. That doesn't mean hanging it up randomly. I am not a fan of randomly programmed workouts where ou are just doing different things everyday. You want a program that you can rogress with, and you have key indicators that you are making progress.

That's exactly what the plan below does. You can use it as a starting point, and tailor it to your needs once you are comfortable. And if you miss a workout once in a while, no big deal- get back on board with your next one and keep going. It is a marathon, not a sprint (unless its HIIT day) but we get to that later.

Here is the basic breakdown of what you'll be doing:

- Strength training three days a week, one hour per session
- High intensity interval training one day a week, 20 minutes per session
- Steady state cardio one day a week, 35 to 45 minutes per session
- Two days of active recovery

Every workout should begin with at least 5 to 10 minutes of warm up. After your workout, make sure you take time to cool down, to relax your nervous system. My favorite thing to do with a client is to lay them down, put their feet up on the wall so that their legs are elevated, and just have them breath into the belly, five second to inhale and five second to exhale, jus to mellow everything out.

After a couple if minuets, stench out your major muscle groups (flexibility increases when muscles are warm), and hold each stretch for at least three breathes.

Strength training- 1 hour (3 days per week)

You may thing you only have to do cardio, cardio if you are trying to loose weight, but strength training is incredibly important because having more muscle mass increases your metabolic rate, which means you, will burn more calories at rest while your body works to maintain muscle tissues.
You will want to do full body-training sessions. Working specific body parts for as full session (like chest and triceps) can be great, but when life happens and you have to miss a workout, your routine and muscles will be imbalance. Hitting all in one training session is a better bet fir most people.

What to do:

- ***Compound lower body exercise (deadlift, squats)***
  Any compound lower body move or variation will work for this one, like a goblet squats or a dumbbell deadlift. A compound movement is one that works multiple muscle groups.The key here is to lift heavy; I am talking about using some of the biggest muscle groups in your body, and in order to get those muscles to respond, you need to challenge them.

There is no set amount of reps or sets for this part of the workout, although I recommend working up to your 5-rep max during every session. This means starting at a weight that is not challenging and working your way up. Do 5 reps with a relatively light weight, rest, do 5 reps with a weight that is 5 pounds heavier, rest, and keep repeating this pattern, using 5 more pounds every time. When you hit a weight where you can only do 5 with good form, you are done- keep that number in mind and try to beat it over.

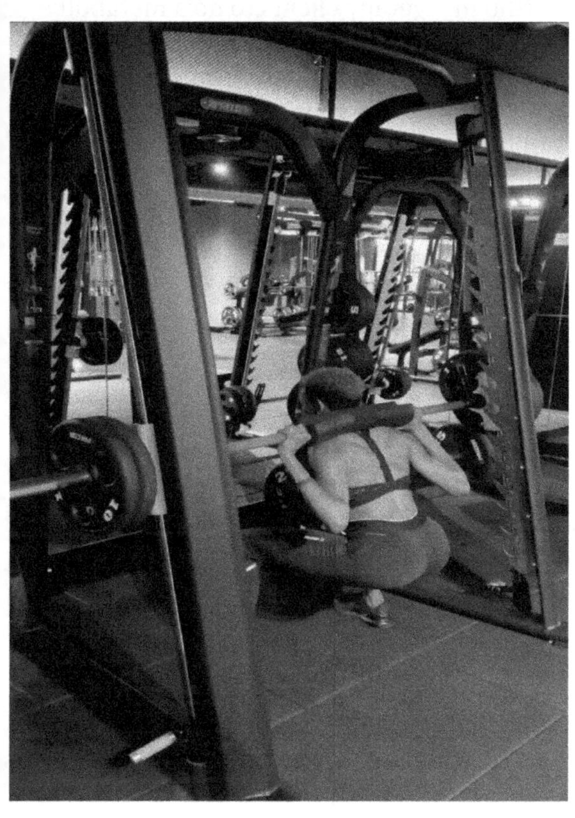

- ***Upper-body supersets: Upper body pushing exercises (dumbbell bench press, push-ups) & Upper body pulling exercises (single arm-bend over row, dumbbell curl)***

You will be super-setting these moves, which means doing one set of the first exercise followed immediately by a set of the other. I recommend doing 3 sets of 12 reps of each move. Don't rest in between two movements (raising your heart rate incorporates some cardio work), but you can take up to 60 seconds break before starting the new set. Alternating between pushing and pulling movements allows you to work opposing muscle groups.

- ***Lower body/core superset: Unilateral lower-body move (reverse lunge, step-up) & core movement (plank, Russian twist)***

A unilateral lower body move is one where you work one leg at a time (another example is the Bulgarian split). By working only one side at a time, you can be sure you are not relying on one leg more than the other. This helps with keeping the muscle imbalance in check. After you have done both sides, you can superset it with an abs movement.

Again do three sets of 12 reps without resting in between the exercises (feel free to take 60 minutes rest between sets). If you choose a plank for the core move, hold for at least 30 seconds.

- ***Metabolic finisher***

This is where you will get a boost of cardio in. I get my clients to do a metabolic finisher at the end of a strength workout to get the heart rate going for more immediate calorie burns. You could choose an exercise and do it for a certain amount of time (say 3 minutes of quickly jumping the rope), or decide to a certain number of a move and finish them as quickly as possible (e.g. Doing 15 burpees as fast as you can). The time you take, and what move you chose is entirely up to you, so mix it up. If you need a starting point, I suggest 10 burpees, 10 mountain climbers and 10 plank ups for seven minutes, trying to do as many rounds as possible (and aiming to beat yourself next time). Then, cool it down and you are done for the day.

The first of your two days of cardio should be high-intensity interval training (HIIT). Steady state cardio does have a place in your routine (we will get there), but don't forget that intensity is your friend. This is going to incite way more fat loss than just steady state cardio. When you are working in that high-intensity threshold, you are not only burning more calories but you raise your metabolic rate significantly afterwards. Your body will need to work harder and longer to return to a resting state, burning more calories in the process.

What to do:

Choose an activity you like as a template- maybe it is running, cycling, or bodyweight moves. Whatever it is, push as hard as you possibly can for 30 seconds then back off for the rest period. How long you rest will depend on your fitness level. If you are just starting out, you may want to try a 2-to-1 rest to work ratio, (so 30 seconds of work followed by 60 seconds of rest). Than you can reduce your rest time every week. You could also try Tabata intervals once you get comfortable – that's 20 seconds of extreme hard work circuit until 20 minutes are up.

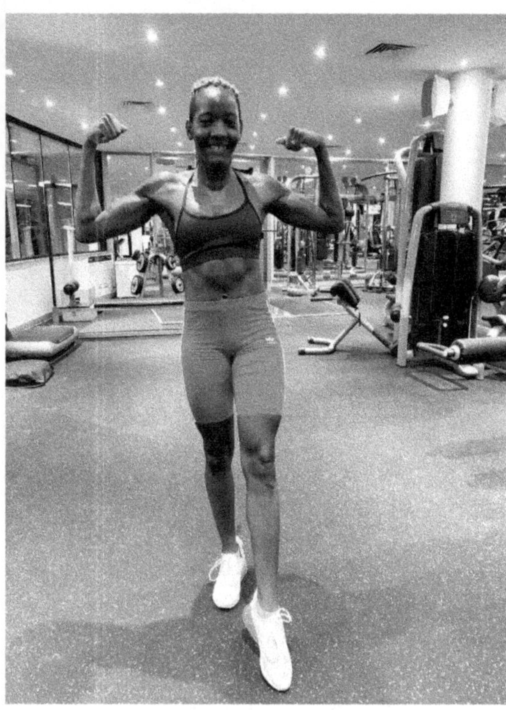

I came up with a 21 days weight loss workouts that you will love and enjoy:

Here is how it works: every week you will do six workouts (none of them lasts more than about half an hour):

- Two total body toning
- Two fat blasting interval workouts
- Two easy recovery session

Total-Body toning Routines- 2x a week
Reps: 12-15 per move
Set: 1 set during week 1, 2 set during week 2 and 3 sets during week 3
Moves
Plank with alternating leg lift
Wood chop with resistance band
Dumbbell Squats with Overhead Press
Romanian Deadlift
Bent-Over Row
Dynamic Lunges
Fat-Blasting Intervals- 2x a week
Do the following three moves back to back with no rest in between. That is one interval.
Rest for one to two minutes between the intervals. Complete as many reps of each move as you can in the prescribed amount of time.

Week 1: 20 seconds per move, 5 intervals
Week 2: 30 seconds per move, 6 intervals
Week 3: 40 seconds per move, 7 intervals

Moves
Mountain Climber
Lateral Shuffle
Jump Squat

Result –Enhancing Recovery- 2x a week
Do the following three moves in the order shown. Repeat two or three times.

Moves:
Hip Flexor Stretch
Double Hip Extension
Standing Chest Stretch
Floor I-position Raise

B) Muscle Growth

You have probably heard that you should be incorporating strength training into your exercise routine. But hitting the weights may feel much more intimidating than taking a walk or jog around your neighborhood.

While results may not always be fast, creating a solid strength training routine should show you noticeable muscle gains in a few weeks to several months.

How does Muscles Grow?

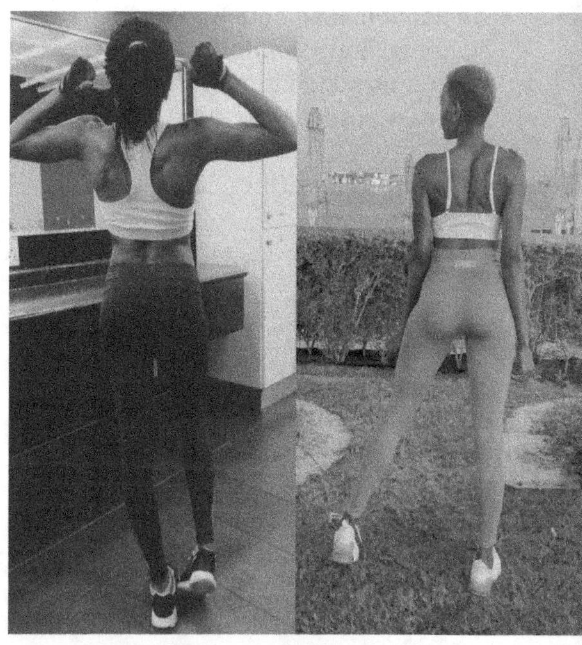

Muscles growth requires three things: Stimulus, fuel and repair. When you do extreme exercises, it makes the muscle work, drains its energy store and causes micro scoping damage to the muscle fibers, or what's called muscle injury. After exercise the muscles must replenish its fuel tank and repair it self. Provided that ne exercise (stimulus) was of sufficient intensity, the muscle will grow during the epair process.

ertain hormones actually help your muscles grow too. They control the satellite ells and are responsible for things like:

- Sending the cells to your muscles after exercise
- Forming new blood capillaries
- Repairing muscle cells
- Managing muscle mass

or example resistance moves help your body release growth hormone from your ituitary gland, how much is released depends on the intensity of the exercise you ave done. Growth hormone triggers your metabolism and helps turn amino acids nto protein to bulk up your muscles.

ow To Build Muscle

pending your whole day in the gym isn't necessary to build muscles. Weight raining 20-30 minutes, 2 to 3 times per week is enough to see results. You should y to target all your major muscle groups at least twice throughout your weekly orkouts.

While you may not see results right away, even a single strength training session an help promote muscle growth. Exercise stimulates what is called Protein ynthesis in 2 to 4 hours after you finish your workout. Your levels may stay levated for up to a whole day.

trength training activities includes:

- Body weight exercises, like push ups, squats and lunges
- Resistance band movements
- Workouts with stationary weight machines, like leg curl machine
- Workouts with free weights such as dumbbells

When you lift, you should try to do between 8 to 15 reps in a row. That is one set. Wait a minute in between sets to rest, than complete another set of the same ength. Take approximately 3 seconds to lift or push your weight into place. Than old that position for a full second and take another slow 3 seconds to lower the eight.

Resistance VS Reps

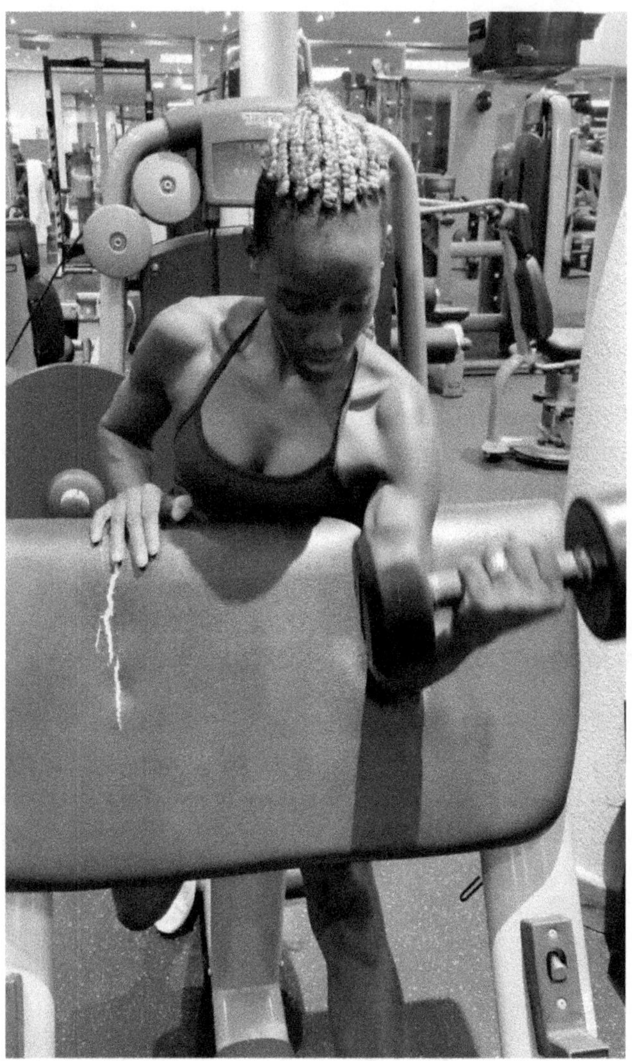

You should aim to lift heavy weight, enough to challenge you. This is known as resistance training. A good example is to select a weight that tires your muscles after 12 to 15 reps. when you can easily do 15 reps on that same weight, than sta to gradually increase the weight to the next level.

Even a single set of 12 reps with a heavy enough weight can help build your muscles more than a 3 sets of lighter weight.

Muscle growth: Man VS Women

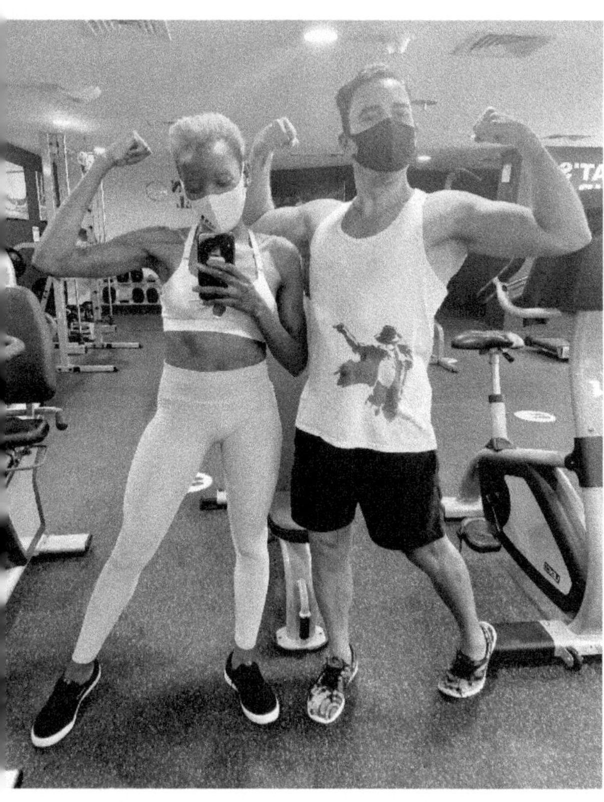

Man and women build muscles differently. This is because testosterone plays a big role in muscle development. While both have testosterones in they're bodies, several studies shown that both men and women have similar response to strength training.

In conclusion, change in muscle mass is more noticeable on both sexes with more muscle mass to begin with.

Cardio and Muscles

Cardio exercising, also known as aerobic, raises your heart and breathing rates. It strengthens your cardiovascular system.

The case that "Cardio isn't too good for building muscles" isn't entirely the case. Cardio exercise can actually help with muscle growth, muscle function and your overall exercise capacity. These effects are particularly noted in older and sedentary individuals.

For cardio exercising to promote muscle growth, it has to be performed at least at the intensity of 70-80 percent heart rate reserve (HRR), 30 to 45 minutes in length, 4 to 5 days a week.

Tips for better Results

1. **Break your fast**

Eating protein for breakfast is one of the best things you can do when wanting to add muscles and burn fat. Protein allows you for a slow ad steady rise in blood sugar levels, which keeps you feeling fuller for longer so you aren't tempted to snack on sweet treats before lunch. It also repairs the damage done to your muscles through training, to rebuild your muscles bigger and stronger after every session.

2. **Load up on veg**

You should be eating protein at every meal, preferably high quality lean source such as teak, chicken, turkey and white fish, but making up most of each meal-about half your plate in fact should be vegetables. That's because it is high in antioxidants and essential vitamins and minerals to keep you fighting fit, and full of fiber to keep you feeling full longer after you eat. Vegetables are also very high in calories. Eat a wide variety of colors for variety of nutrients.

3. **Time your Carbs**

For the duration of this workout plan you should cut back on your carbs intake, especially heavily processed cards such as crisps, chips and white bread and pasta. But you still need carbs to help you recover from training, and it is important to be fully energized for each session so you can push yourself. Stick to cards in their natural form, such as potatoes or whole meal rice. Eta them around your workouts, then back off for the rest of the day.

4. **Drink more water**

If you are dehydrated, your body is going to have a tough time both building new muscles mass and burning fat stores. And dehydration results in poor focus and lack of motivation, which will make it much harder to get to the gym and train well, as well as to make smart nutrition choices. Drink two to three liters a day, but more on training days, to stay hydrated and keep your body looking and feeling in optimal nick.

5. **Eat Enough Protein**

It is easy to get carried away and start gulping down protein shakes several times a day when you are trying to build muscles, but while you will need an increase in protein, you don't need to go overboard. If you are just stating to strength train you will probably hit your daily protein intake (1.2-2 g per body weight per day) easily, just but changing your diet slightly, thought supplements can also be also be useful.

Three weeks Muscle Gain Training Plan

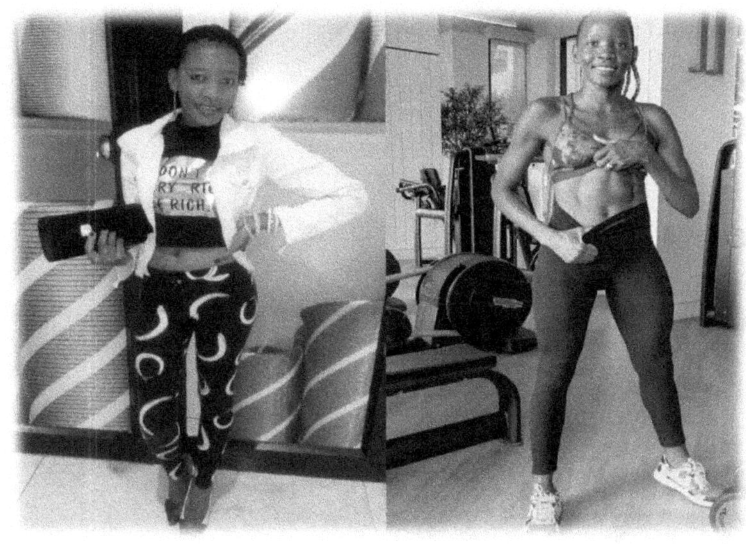

This plan has four sessions a week: Chest and Arms; Legs and Shoulder; Back and Arms; and Chest and Shoulders. This way you will train all your major upper-body muscles directly or indirectly twice a week, an intensive approach that will add muscle fast.

The first week of this plan, as you know, it isn't easy, but it is effective. Because the only way to add on lean muscle mass quickly while also stripping away unwanted belly fat is to push your muscles harder with enough high quality reps, and with only the briefest rest between sets and moves to keep your heart rate high.

In the second and third week of the plan, you will do the same workouts in the same order as the first week. However, while the total number of sets and reps for move one and two remain the same, there is an extra set for all the other moves in the workout. This means you will do a total of five sets for moves 3, 4 and a superset for 5, up from four total sets in the week 1.

If possible, try to lift slightly heavier weights than in the previous week, especially for the first two moves, and at least the first set or two of all subsequent moves. Even a small increase, so long as your form doesn't suffer, will add up to a big difference to your progress.

Monday Workout: Chest and Back

Exercises	Sets	Reps	Tempo	Rest (Sec)
Bench press	4	8	2010	60
Lat Pull Down	4	8	2011	60
Cable Cross Over	4	12	2010	60
Declined Dumbbell Press	4	12	2011	30
Rope Face Pulls	4	12	2010	60

Bench press
*(*Chest, triceps)

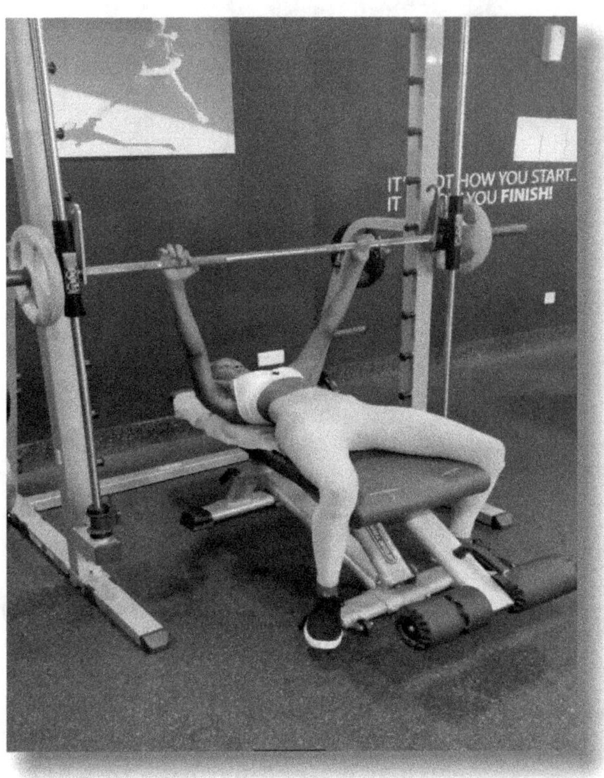

- ***Tips***:
- Lie back on a flat bench holding a barbell in the rack above you with a shoulder-width, overhand grip.
- Drive your feet into the floor to contract your quads and glutes, and clamp back your shoulder blades to shorten the weight's path of travel. This increases neural drive to your chest, delts and triceps.
- From the starting position, breathe in and lower the bar slowly until it skims the middle of your chest.
- Focus your mind on activating your chest muscles and push the bar back to the starting position explosively as you breathe out. That's one rep, repeat as desired.

at Pull Down:
-ats, shoulders***)***

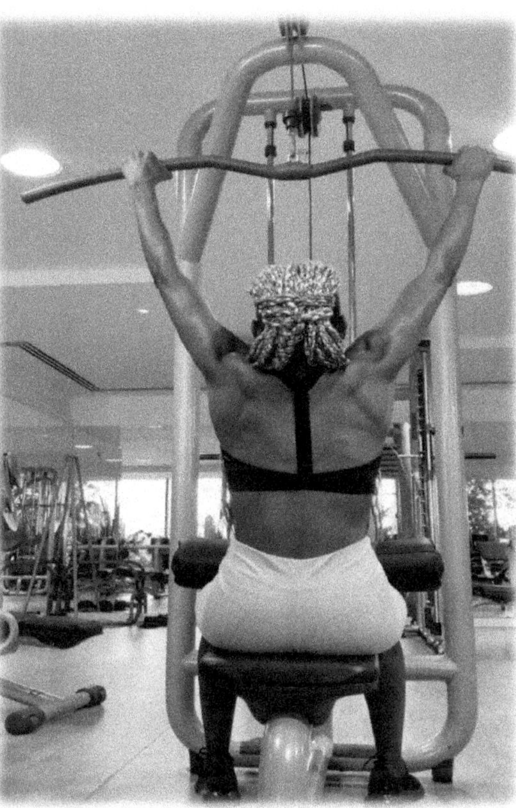

'ips:

- Grasp the bar with a wide grip with an overhand, knuckles-up grip. Other positions and grips are possible, but start with this standard position.
- Pull the bar down until it's approximately level with the chin. Exhale on the downward motion. While shifting just slightly backward is OK, aim to keep your upper torso stationary. Keep your feet flat on the floor and engage your abs as you pull. The bottom of the motion should be where your elbows can't move downward any more without moving backward. Be sure to stop at that point and do not go lower.
- Squeeze the shoulder blades together while maintaining square shoulders.
- From the bottom position, with the bar close to your chin, slowly return the bar to the starting position while controlling its gradual ascent. Don't let it crash into the weight plates.

Cable Cross Overs:
*(*Pectorales/Chest*)*

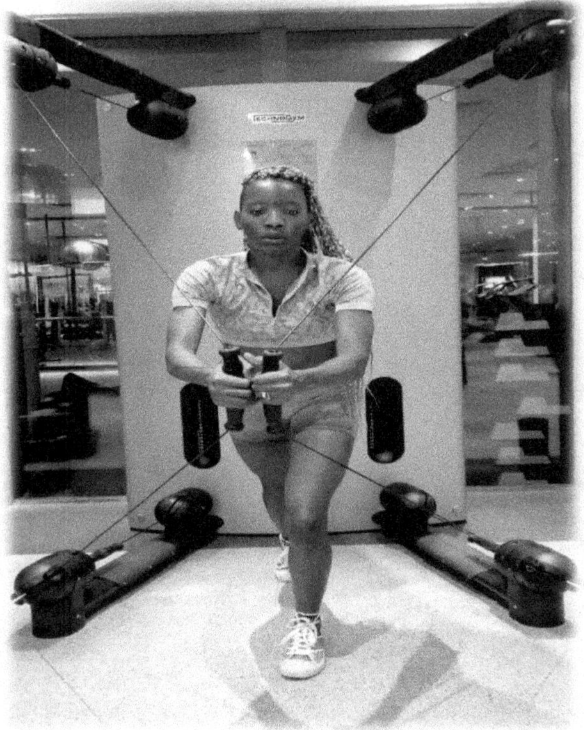

Tips:

- Take one in each hand – your arms should be outstretched with a slight bend.
- Place one foot slightly in front of the other, and slightly lean forward.
- To start, place the pulleys on a high position, select the resistance you war to use and hold the pulleys in each hand. Step forward between both pulleys, while pulling your arms together in front of you and slightly bending the torso forward.

Decline Dumbbell Press
(Pecs, Delts and Triceps*)*

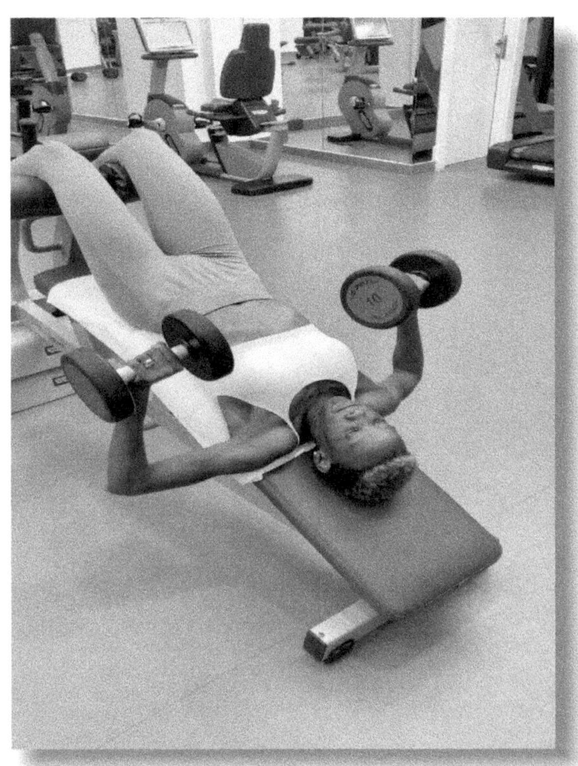

Tips:

- Tuck your feet firmly between the pads, with each dumbbell on your knees. Lie back on the bench and bring the dumbbells back to your chest and push up as you lay down.
- Squeeze your shoulder blades by pinching them together and driving them into the bench and slightly arch your back.
- Make sure your palms are rotated completely under the dumbbells, squeezing them tight.
- As you descend, follow your bend your elbows at a parallel 90 degrees, then push back up bringing the dumbbells together, while still keeping a slight bend in your elbows, not locking out.

Rope face pulls
*(*Traps and Upper back*)*

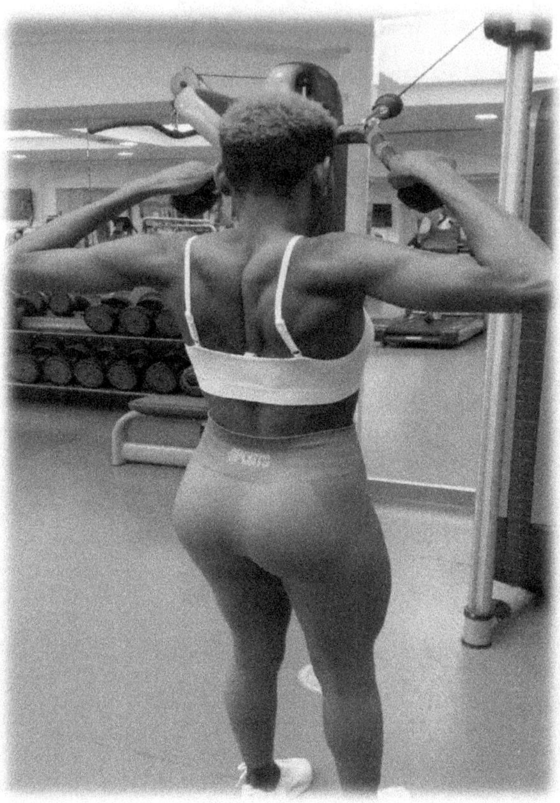

Tips:

- Stand facing the cable machine and grab the ends of the rope with each hand. Use an underhand grip right above the ball end, with your thumbs facing you.
- Maintain an athletic stance throughout your reps. Feet hip- to shoulder-width apart, slight bend to the knees, core engaged to keep your upper body steady. If a split stance is more comfortable, then use it.
- Position the ropes so that the cable is taught, but the weight hasn't lifted yet. Your arms should be face height and straight out in front of you.
- Begin by squeezing your shoulder blades and bringing the rope back towards your face.
- Continue to pull the rope back, allowing your hands to move past your ears before your elbows.
- Keep pulling the rope until your hands are past your ears, but before the rope reaches your face.
- Squeeze your shoulders for a second or two before you move your hands back to the starting position.

Wednesday Workout: Legs and Cardio

Exercises	Sets	Reps	Tempo	Rest (Sec)
Barbell Squats	4	8	2010	60
Wide stance squats	4	8	2011	60
Leg Extension	4	12	2010	60
Hamstring curl	4	12	2011	30
Bulgarian splits	4	12	2010	60

Barbell Squats
*(*Lower body Muscles*)*

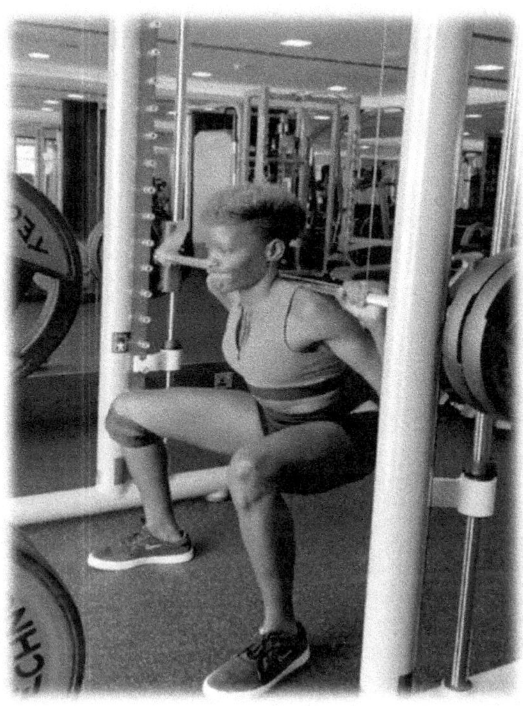

Tips:

- Set up a barbell to the appropriate height in the squat rack according to your height. The barbell should be slightly lower than your shoulders. Make sure you have enough space to take a couple of steps backward after unracking the barbell.
- While facing the barbell, step underneath the barbell and place your hands on both sides of it. The barbell should rest on the muscles of your upper back.
- Keep your posture tall, with your feet slightly wider than hip-width apart and a slight bend in your knees. Your shoulders should be directly over your hips with a neutral head and neck position. Your chin should remain tucked throughout the movement as if you were holding an egg under your chin.

- Pre-tension your shoulders and hips, and engage your core. Your ribs should be down and your pelvis should be slightly tucked.
- While maintaining your alignment, begin the downward movement by bending your hips, knees, and ankles.
- Lower until your legs are parallel or slightly below parallel to the floor. Keep your weight evenly distributed on your feet as you lower.
- Pause for a second at the bottom position.
- To begin the upward movement, push your feet into the ground to initiate standing up. Emphasize pushing through your midfoot and heel while keeping your toes engaged.
- As you begin to stand up, keep your chest high, squeeze your glutes, and allow your knees to straighten and your hips to travel forward.
- As you finish the movement, squeeze your glutes and quadriceps while maintaining a neutral spine.

Wide Stance Squats
*(*Adductors, Hamstrings, Glutes*)*

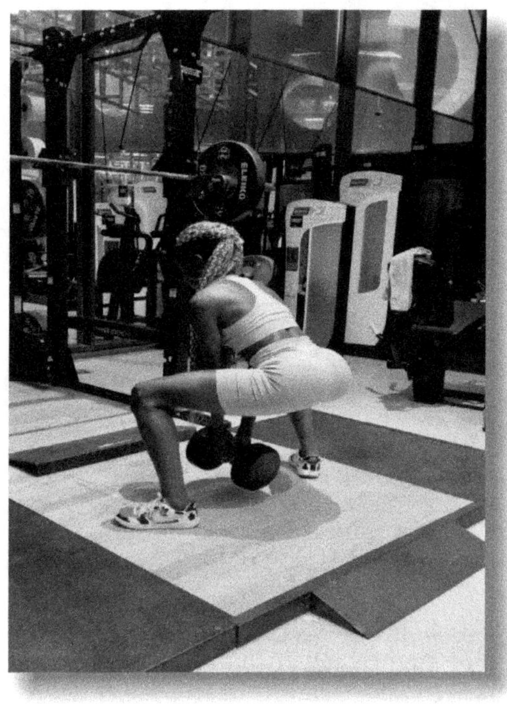

Tips:

- Stand with feet wider than shoulders, knee slightly bent, toes turned outward. Hold a dumbbell with both hands in front of body.
- INHALE: Squat until thighs are nearly parallel to the floor, sticking butt out as if sitting in a chair.
- EXHALE: Squeeze glutes as you straighten legs to starting position to complete one rep.
- Keep your core braced and make sure your knees don't pass the line of toes.

- ***Leg Extension***
  *(*Quads*)*

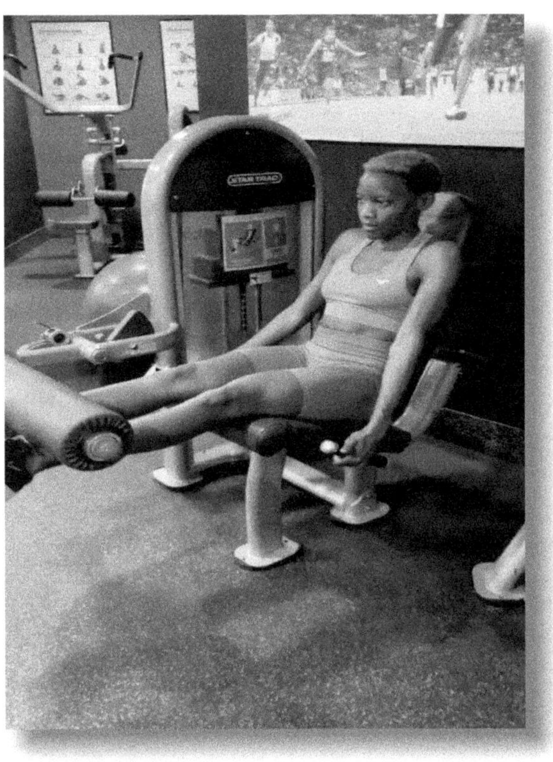

Tips:

- Set up the leg extension machine so the pad is at the top of your lower legs at the ankles. Your knees are at 90 degrees.
- Place your hands on the hands bar
- Lift the weight while exhaling until your legs are almost straight. Do not lock your knees. Keep your back against the backrest and do not arch your back

Hamstring Curl
*(*Hamstrings, Calf muscle*)*

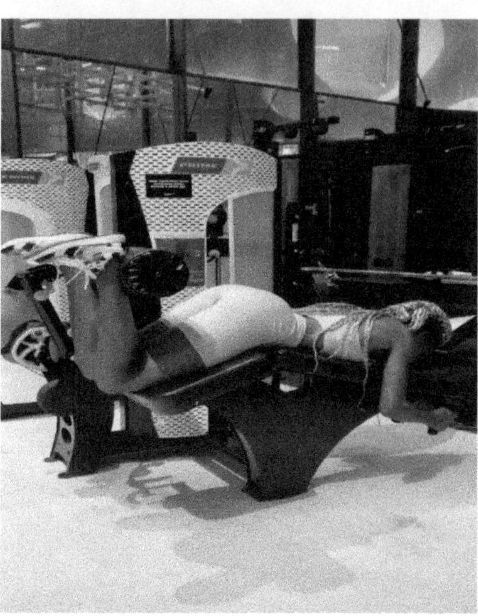

Tips:

- Lie down on the leg curl machine, stretching your legs out fully. The roller pad should rest a few inches over your calves, just above the heels. Hold th support handles on each side of the machine.
- Exhale and flex your knees, pulling your ankles as close to your buttocks as you can. Keep your hips firmly on the bench
- Inhale as you return your feet to the starting position in a slow and controlled movement.

Bulgarian Splits
*(*Quads, hamstrings, Calves*)*

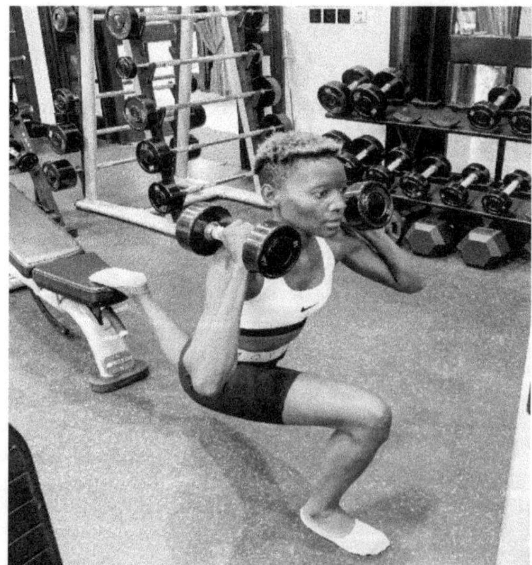

Tips:

- Rest your back foot on a bench about knee height
- Get into a forward lunge position with torso upright, core braced and hips square to your body, with your back foot elevated on the bench. Your leading leg should be half a meter or so in front of the bench.
- Lower until your thigh is almost horizontal, keep your knee in line with your foot. Don't let your front knee travel beyond your toes.
- Drive up through your front heel back to the starting position, again keeping your movement measured.

Cardio (10-15 Minutes)

Exercises	Time
Daedmill Sprint	30 Secs
Active rest:	60 Secs
Burpees	
Jump rope	

Dead mill Sprint

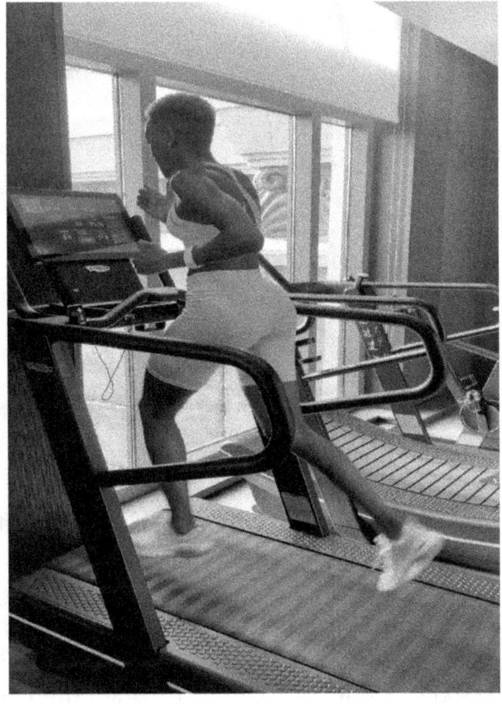

Friday Workout: Arms

Exercises	Sets	Reps	Tempo	Rest (Sec)
Triceps push down	4	10	2010	60
Cable Curl	4	10	2011	60
Overhead dumbbell extension	4	12	2010	60
Inclined Bicep curls	4	12	2011	30
Triceps Dips	4	12	2010	60

Triceps push down
*(*Triceps*)*

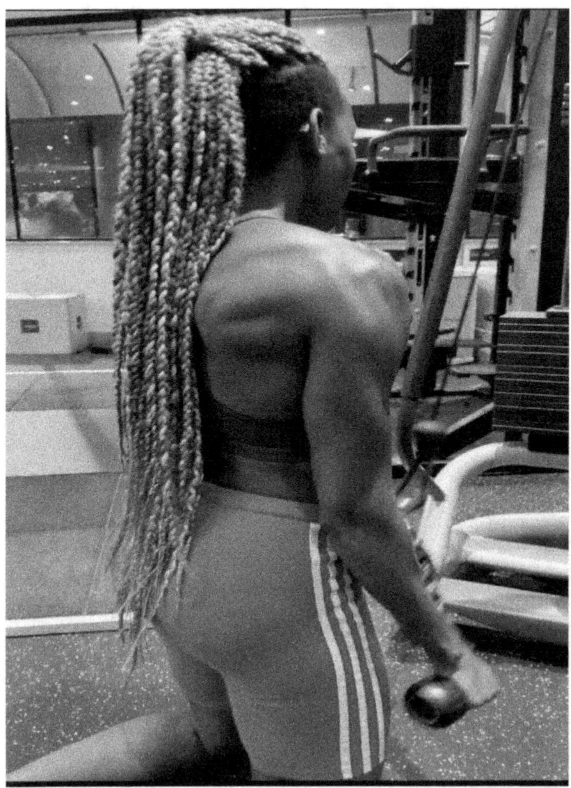

Tips:

- Tilt your torso forward at 30-40 degree angel instead of standing straight up, or modified perform it on your knees
- From this stance, grip the rope as you normally would and pull it down until your upper arm forms a 90-degree angle with your sides. That's your starting point.
- From there, drive your arms down until your entire arm is perpendicular to the floor. That's the bottom of the rep.
- The forward lean is allowing all three triceps heads to move through their full range of motion.

Cable curl
*(*Biceps*)*

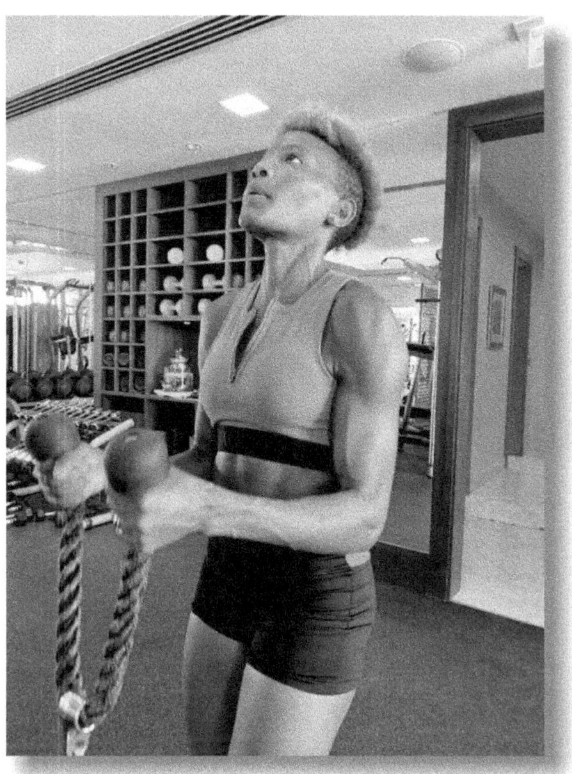

Tips:

- Place a rope attachment on a low pulley and stand facing the machine. You should be about 12 inches away from it.
- Grasp the rope with a palms-in grip. Stand straight up while keeping the natural arch of your back and torso stationary.
- Pull your elbows in to your side and keep them in position during the entire exercise. This is the starting position for the exercise.
- Use your biceps to pull your arms up until your biceps touch your forearms. Exhale as you do so.
- Stop for a second at the top and hold for a second while squeezing your biceps, then slowly bring your weight back to the original position.
- Repeat the process for the desired number of repetitions.

Overheard Dumbbell extension
*(*Triceps*)*

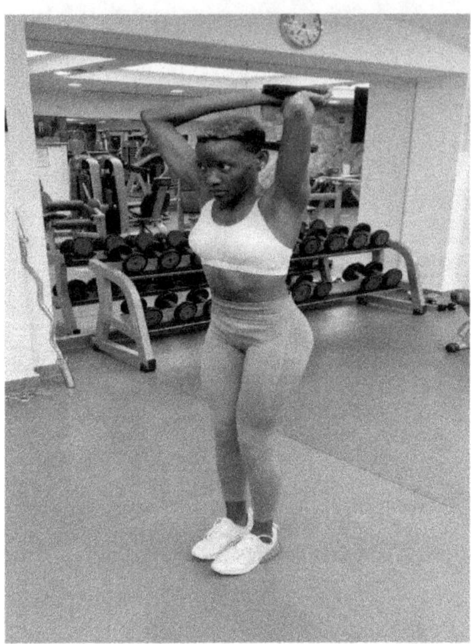

Tips:

- Start standing with your feet shoulder width apart and dumbbells held in front of you.
- Raise the dumbbells above your head until your arms are stretched out straight. Slowly lower the weights back behind your head, being careful not to flare your elbows out too much.
- Once your forearms move beyond parallel to the floor bring the weight back up to the starting position. Your upper arms should remain in place throughout the movement.

Inclined Bicep curls
*(*Biceps*)*

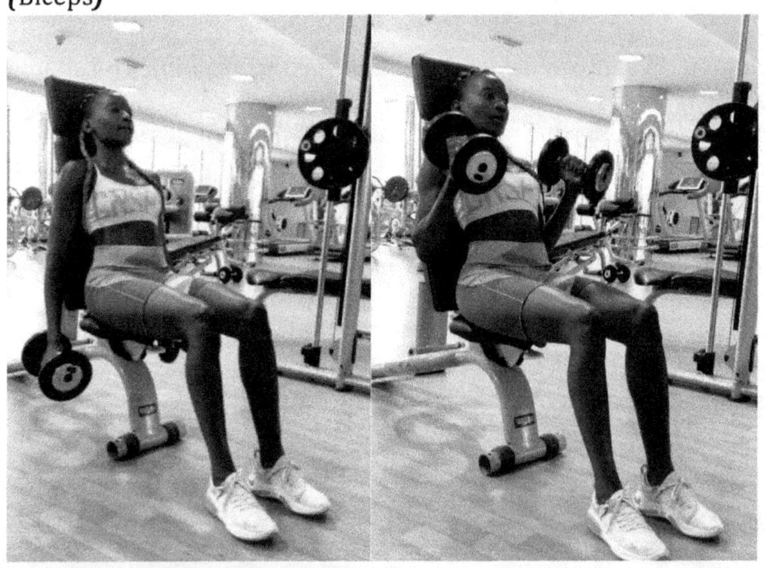

ips:

- Start by adjusting the bench so that it inclines to about 45 degrees. Place the dumbbells on the sides of the bench.
- Proceed to sit on the bench. Grab the dumbbells on both hands and suspend them on your sides ensuring that your elbows are close to your torso. Keep your back straight on the inclined pad and press your feet firmly on the floor. Ensure that you engage your core throughout the entire exercise. This marks your starting position.
- Curl both hands simultaneously ensuring that you bring the weights close to your armpits. Exhale and contract your biceps while doing this. Ensure that your palms should face upwards.
- Pause briefly then lower the dumbbells to your starting position in a slow and controlled motion.

Triceps Dips
*(*Triceps*)*

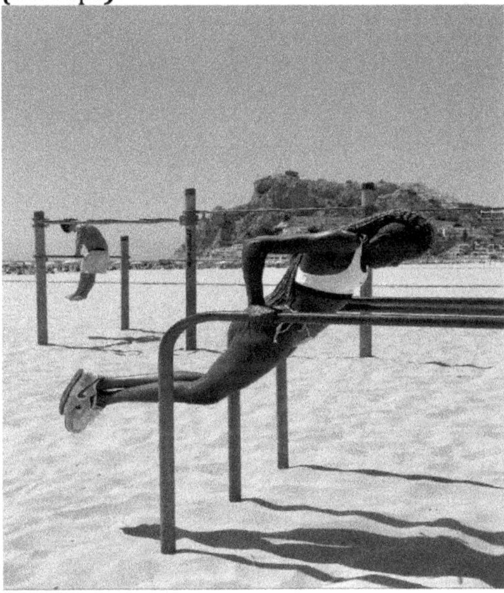

Tips:

- Grab the parallel bars and lift yourself up until arms are fully extended.
- Let your thighs hang downward, bend your knees slightly and hook one foot over the other.
- From this start position, bend your elbows and slowly lower your body until your upper arms are parallel to the floor.
- Keep your torso upright and your elbows close to your sides. Pause momentarily in the bottom position then push yourself back up until your elbows lock out.
- Contract your triceps forcefully

Sunday Workout: Shoulder and abs

Exercises	Sets	Reps	Tempo	Rest (Sec)
Alternating overhead press	4	10	2010	60
Upright row	4	10	2011	60
Dumbbell shrugs	4	12	2010	60
Front raise (W/plate)	4	12	2011	30
High Pulley Lateral extensions	4	12	2010	60

Alternating Overheard press

*(*Shoulders, anterior delts, arms*)*

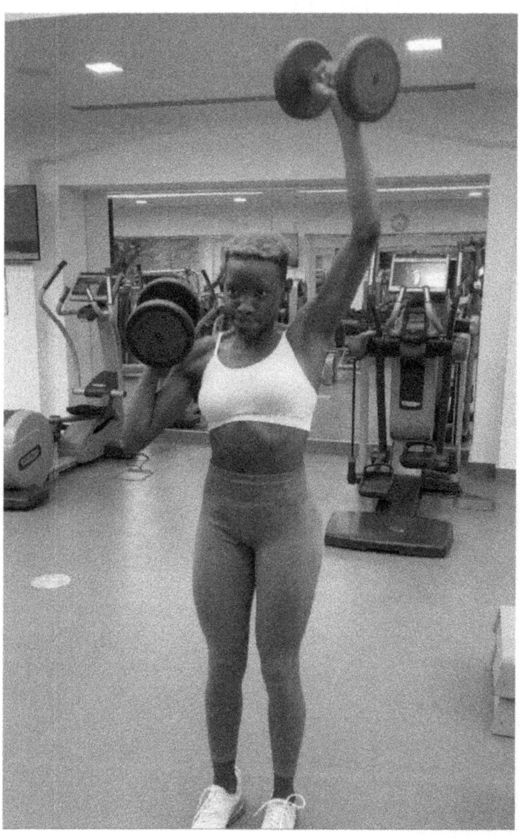

Tips:

- Holding a dumbbell in each hand, plant both feet on the floor hip-width apart. Extend both arms overhead, holding the dumbbells in an overhand grip (palms facing away from your body). This is your starting position.
- Inhale. Without moving your left arm, bend your right elbow to lower the dumbbell down to chin height.
- Exhale. Using the muscles in your shoulder and arm, extend your right elbow to return to the starting position. Avoid "shrugging" by drawing your shoulder blades down and back.
- Inhale. Without moving your right arm, bend your left elbow to lower the dumbbell down to chin height.
- Exhale. Using the muscles in your shoulder and arm, extend your left elbow to return to the starting position. Once again, avoid "shrugging" by drawing

your shoulder blades down and back. Continue alternating between right and left for the specified number of repetitions.

Upright Row
*(*Shoulders, Upper back*)*

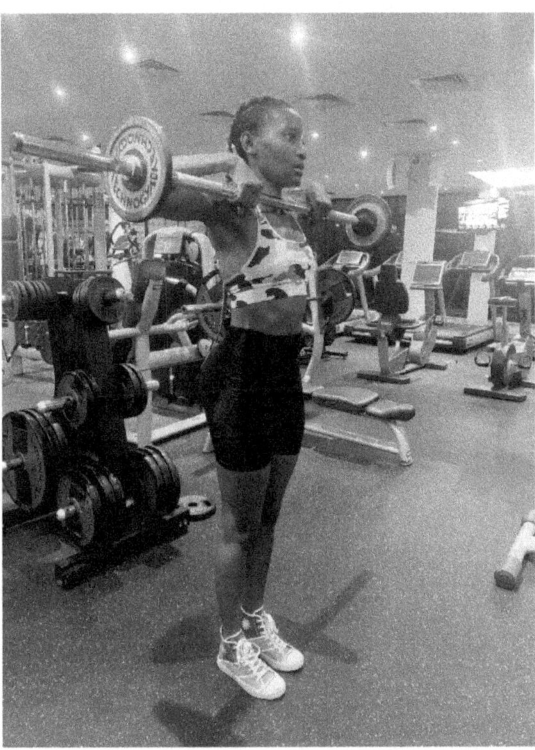

Tips:

- Breathe in and brace the abdominal. Keep your back straight, chest up, and eyes focused forward.
- Lift the barbell straight up (toward the chin) as you exhale. Lead with the elbows and keep the bar close to the body. Your arms should go no higher than parallel with the shoulders; slightly less is okay.
- Pause at the top of the lift.
- Lower the barbell as you inhale, returning it to the starting position.

Dumbbell Shrugs
*(*Shoulders, Traps and Forearms*)*

Tips:

- Grab a pair of dumbbells and hold them by your sides. Your palms should be facing your legs. Your posture should be tall, with your feet shoulder-width apart and a slight bend in your knees. Your shoulders should be directly over your hips with a neutral head and neck position. Your arms should remain long by your sides, with a slight bend in your elbows. Your chin should remain tucked throughout the movement as if you were holding an egg under your chin.

- Grip the floor with your feet to create a stable foot position. Evenly distribute your weight along the length of your feet.
- 3. Pre-tension your shoulders, hips, and engage your core. Your ribs should be down, and you should slightly tuck your pelvis.
- 4. While maintaining a neutral head and neck position, keep your arms long and slowly raise your shoulders straight up toward your ears.
- 5. Pause for a second at the top of the movement.
- 6. Slowly lower your shoulders back to the starting position.

Front Raises (with Plate)
*(*Shoulders*)*

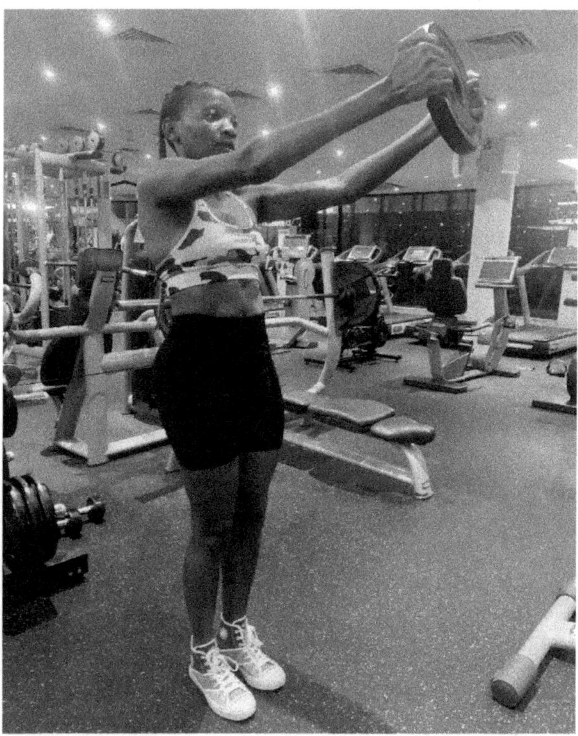

Tips:

- : Stand up straight holding a barbell plate with both hands. They should be positioned at the 3 o'clock and 9 o'clock positions. Your palms should be facing each other and your arms should be extended with your elbows slightly bent. Hold the plate down near your waist. This is the starting position for the exercise.
- Raise the plate until it is slightly above shoulder level. Hold the contraction for a second.
- Bring the plate back to the starting position, inhaling as you do so.
- Repeat for the number of reps in your set

High Pulley Lateral Extension:
(Shoulders***)***

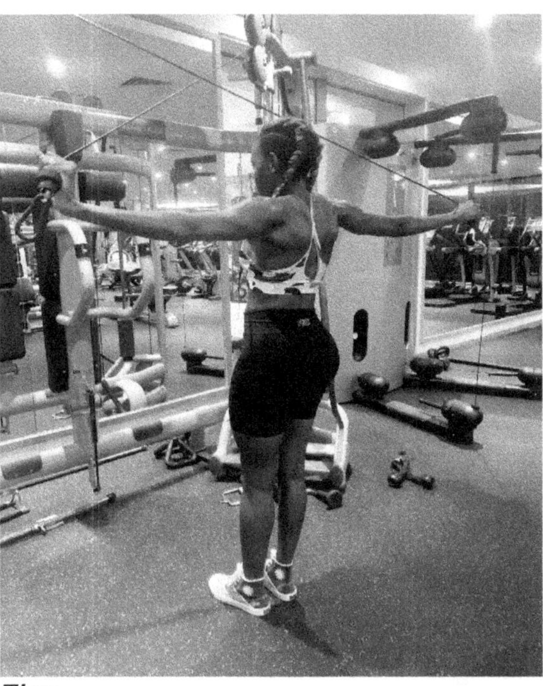

Tips:

- Adjust the pulleys to the appropriate height and adjust the weight. The pulleys should be above your head.
- Grab the left handle with your right hand and the right handle with your left hand. Your arms will start in this crossed position.
- With a tight core, contract your rear delts to bring your arms backward until you feel a pinch in your shoulder blades.
- Slowly bring your arms back to the starting position. You should maintain only a slight bend in your arms during this motion and repeat.

ABS Workout

Exercises	Sets	Reps	Rest (Sec)
Plank with Plate/Dumbbell drag	3	20	60
Weighted Crunches with plate	3	20	60
Bicycle Crunch	3	20	60
Plank Shoulder Taps	3	20	30

Plank with Plate/Dumbbell Drag

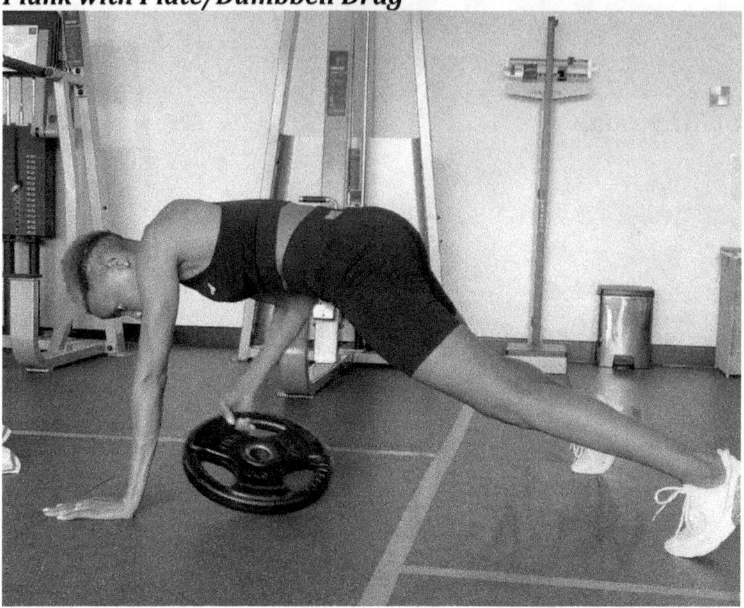

Tips:

- Position yourself in a plank with the plate to the right side of your body.
- With your left hand, reach under the chest and drag the plate to the left side of the body.
- Switch hands, and continue to drag the plate from the right to left side.
- Repeat for desired reps.

Weighted Crunches

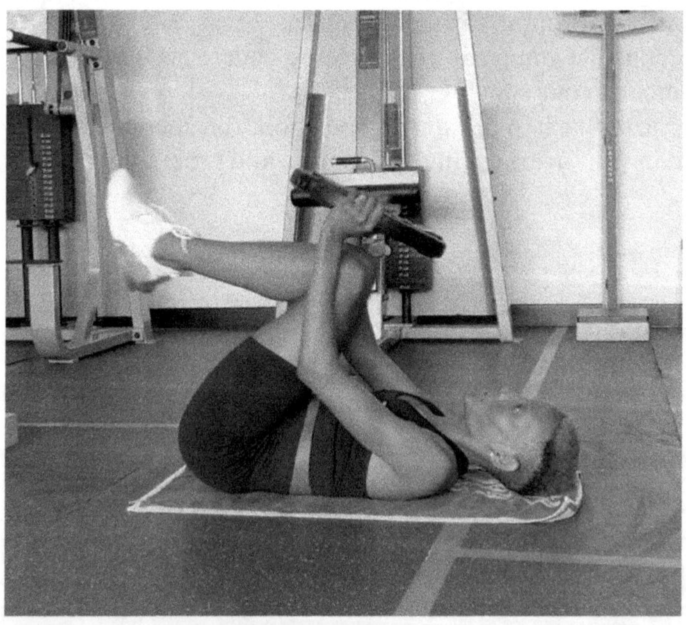

'ips:

- Lay supine in a relaxed position with your knees bent.
- Hold a weight plate directly over your chest and press it to extension.
- Raise your knees to 90 degrees, at which point they will be perpendicular to the floor.
- Exhale as you reach towards your toes with the weight plate.
- Once your abs are fully contracted and your upper back is off the floor, slowly lower yourself back to the starting position.
- Complete for the assigned number of repetitions.

icycle Crunch

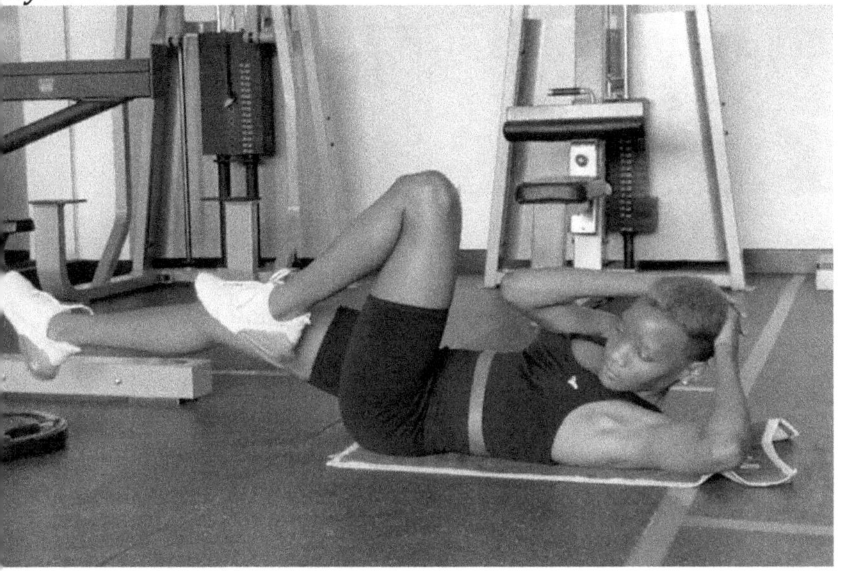

'ips:

- Lie flat on the floor with your lower back pressed to the ground and knees bent. Your feet should be on the floor and your hands are behind your head.
- Contract your core muscles, drawing in your abdomen to stabilize your spine.
- With your hands gently holding your head, pull your shoulder blades back and slowly raise your knees to about a 90-degree angle, lifting your feet from the floor.
- Exhale and slowly, at first, go through a bicycle pedal motion, bringing one knee up towards your armpit while straightening the other leg, keeping both elevated higher than your hips.
- Rotate your torso so you can touch your elbow to the opposite knee as it comes up.
- Alternate to twist to the other side while drawing that knee towards your armpit and the other leg extended until your elbow touches the alternate knee.

Plank Shoulder Taps:

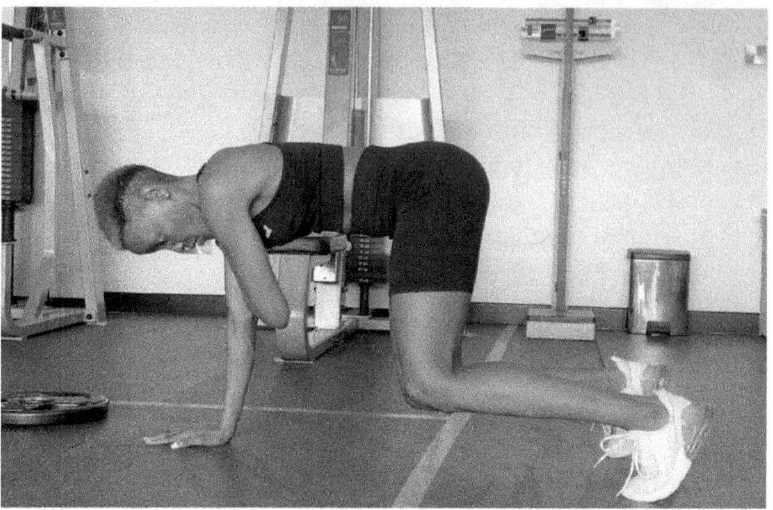

Tips:

- To perform this exercise, start in a press up position and make sure your hands up directly under your shoulders.
- Slightly bend your knees (modified) or keep them straight in line with your hips.
- Keeping your hips as still as posible, lift one hand and tap it on the opposite shoulder. Repeat on the other side.
- Keep repeating this while keeping your body still and tighten your core.

6. Nutrition

<u>Do you need to evaluate your diet?</u>

Yes. If you do not address nutrition, you are missing the foundation of fitness. You cannot out exercise a bad diet. To reap the full rewards of the training program, workout regularly and optimize your nutrition.

Eat meat and vegetable, nuts and seeds, some fruits, little starch and no sugar. Keep intake to level that will support exercise but not body fat. These statement captures a nutritional approach that, when applied with workouts, yields incredible health and fitness. By combining the work potent stimulus of consistency varied functional movements executed at high intensity with a sound diet of whole unprocessed food eaten in the proper amounts, the results are nothing short of life changing.

To truly optimize health and fitness, you have to pay attention to what you eat and how much you eat. That starts with choosing high quality, unprocessed foods and weighting, measuring and recording your intake. I suggest doing that for at least 30 days, you should assess your results, for example: how are your health markers, such as body composition, resting heart rate, and blood pressure (among others)? How are your workouts score trending? How do you feel? From that you can adjust what and how much you are eating for best results.

This type of measured systematic self-observation driven by real results will be the best guide as to whether you should change any of your eating habits or implement any new diet strategies.

Overall, diet needs to be customized to each individual based on their physiological response, goals and other lifestyle factors. The best way to optimize your diet for your specific needs is by carefully tracking inputs (the food you eat) and outputs (workout results and health markers).

7. Rest and Recovery

<u>What is recovery?</u>

One of the most important elements of performances and exercise is rest, and it is also one of the hardest things to do. According to ACE (a fitness governing body), recovery is the most important part of any person's program. Taking time to rest your body can be challenging mentally, but rest has significant physical benefits.

<u>The Recovery Stages</u>

To get better at a sport or to enhance your personal fitness, you must expose your body to stresses. Different stresses include training and exercise programs like weightlifting, sprinting, endurance runs, etc. But upon completion of these stresses the human body needs to adapt to the stresses it just underwent, and this is where we get the recovery stage.

Neglecting the recovery stage can lead to injuries. Many programs have built-in rest days, but if you are creating your own program to follow, make sure to find where to fit one in your routine. It is essential to listen to your body and gauge how you are feeling as well. If you are physically worn out, take a rest.

Benefits of a Rest Day

Rest days are critical for fitness at all levels. Getting adequate rest has both physiological and physiological benefits.

1. Promotes Muscle Recoveries

Exercise depletes the body's stores, or muscle glycogen. It also causes muscle tissue to break down. Giving adequate muscle recovery time allows the body to fix both of these issues; replenishing energy stores and repairing damaged tissues.

If you don't allow sufficient time off to replenish your glycogen stores and give your muscle time to recover from damage, performance will be compromised. Further disregard of replenishment can lead to sustain muscle soreness and pain.

2. **Helps Overcome Adaptation**

The principle adaptation states that when we undergo the stress of physical exercise, our body adapts and becomes more efficient. It is just like learning any new skills. At first, it's difficult, but over time it becomes second nature. Once you adapt to a given stress, you require additional stress to continue to make progress.

But there are limits to how stress the body can tolerate before it breaks down and suffer injury. Doing too much work too quickly will result in injury or muscle damage. Doing too little too slowly will not result in any improvement. This is why personal trainers set up specific programs that increases time and intensity at a planned rate and allows rest days.

3. **Prevents Overtraining**

Too little rest and too few recovery days can lead to overtraining syndrome. This condition is though to affect roughly 60% of elite athletes and 30% of non-elite endurance athletes. And once you have it, it can be difficult to recover.

The consequences of overtraining are many. Research has found that it can increase your body fat, raise your risk of dehydration, lower your libido, and worsen mood.

4. **Promotes Relaxation**

Taking a rest day gives your mind and body a break, and it keeps your schedule from becoming too crowded. Use your free day to spend more time with family and friends. Take your normal exercise time slot and do a hobby instead.

Creating a healthy life is all about balance. It involves finding a way to split your time between home, work and your fitness routine. Taking a rest day allows you to tent to these other areas while giving your body the time it needs to fully recover from your exercise sessions.

What to do on Rest day

Passive recovery

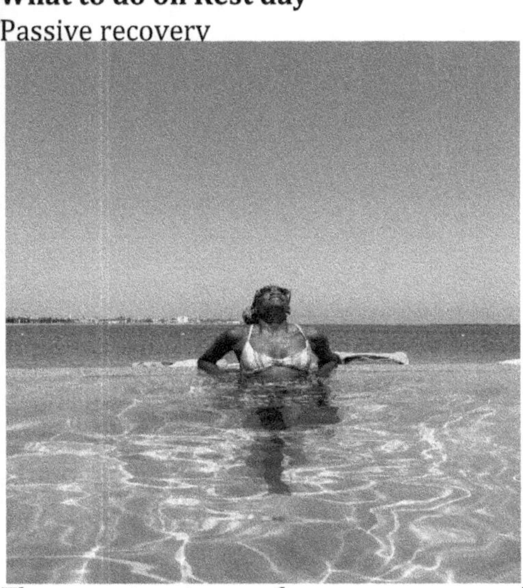

There are two types of recovery you can do on arrest day: passive recovery and active recovery. Passive recovery involves taking the day entirely off from exercise, and active recovery is when you engage in a low intensity exercise, placing minimal stress on the body.

During active recovery, the body works to repair soft tissues (muscle, tendons and ligaments). Active recovery improves blood circulation that helps with the removal of waste products from muscle breakdown that build up as a results of exercise. Then fresh blood can come in to bring nutrients that help repair and re build the muscles. Examples of active recovery exercises include walking, stretching, yoga or even cycling.

Active Recovery

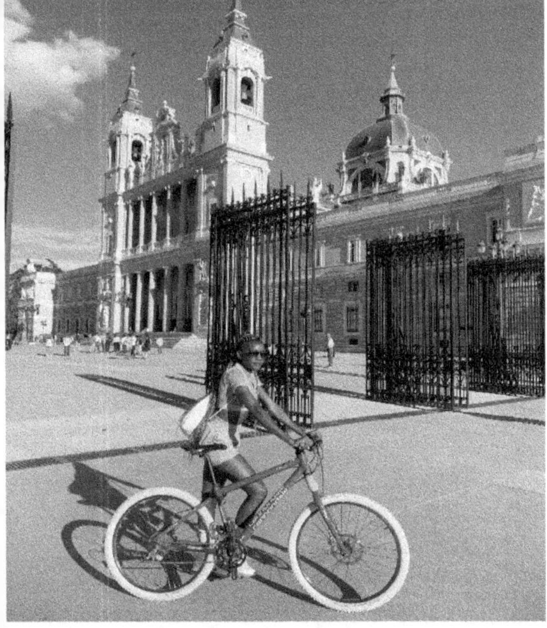

Sleep is important. Make sure to get plenty of rest, especially if you are training hard. Even one or two nights of poor sleep can decrease performance for long bouts of exercise, but not peak performance. However, consistent, inadequate sleep can result in hormone level changes, particularly those related to stress. Research indicates that sleep deprivation can lead to increased levels of cortisol (a stress hormone), decreases activity of human growth hormone, (which is important for tissue repair), and decreased glycogen synthesis.

tarting Tips

ake action: Now that you have read this book, you have the knowledge to start orking on your body. Knowledge is important but now it's the time to walk the alk. It's time to turn your thoughts into action. Actions speak louder than words.

elieve in yourself: Believe to achieve. Everyone has potential; you just have to ake it happen. Believe in yourself and your capabilities.

onsistency: Nothing happens overnight. It takes great willpower to stick with an xercise program and change your dietary habits, but you have to stick with it. You ave to be consistent and patient. Great things take time.

iscipline: We are all creatures of habit. T build a better body, you need to make ight adjustments to your to your daily routine. You have to squeeze in that 30 inutes workout and stick to healthy diet.

volution: Your body evolves and you have to change with it. You will become ronger and fitter. It's all about progress. If you are not making any progress, take step back to evaluate it. Fix the problem and keep moving.

rogress: To make sure you are moving in the right direction towards your goals, ou need to track your progress. You need to know where you are at and if you are etting any results.

inal Tips: Enjoy and have fun. To be doing something for longer, you need to njoy it. Bring your mind around it to get yourself used to it. Choose exercises that ou enjoy the most, join a gym with a good atmosphere, train with a motivated orkout buddy and don't be scared to ask for help.

Appendix 1

Food Nutrition Facts

Food	Protein	Carbohydrates	Fat	Calories
Chicken breast (170g)	35	0	6	200
Lean Beef (170g)	35	0	6	200
Turkey Breast (170g)	35	0	3	180
Tuna (water packed) (170g)	35	0	2	160
Egg white (1)	6	0	0	24
Non fat Milk (240 ml)	9	12	0	90
Rice (50g)	3	39	0	170
Pasta (50g)	6	40	1	200
Potato (1 Medium)	2	35	0	160
Oats (40g)	5	27	3	150
Carrots (80g)	1	9	0	40
Broccoli (80g)	1	4	0	20
Spinach (80g)	2	3	0	20
Whole Wheat bread (1 slice)	4	18	2	110
Low fat Granola	4	36	4	200

Values are approximate. Check the nutrition fact labeling on individual brands. These food are future is the sample meal plans below.

Muscle Mass Sample Meal Plan

Breakfast	Egg white scramble: Mix five egg whites and half a york with a tablespoon of non-milk fat. Cook in a nonstick pan coated with nonfat cooking spray. Serve on two slices of whole-wheat toast. Take with a cup of black coffee or water. **Calories:** 350
Mid morning Snack	Meal Replacement drink: Mix one sachet of a meal replacement powder with 12 oz. cold water in a blender. **Calories:** 340
Lunch	Beef Meal: Cook 6 oz. of lean ground beef in a non-stick pan. Drain excess fat and water. Mix with steamed chopped carrots. Serve with one portion of pasta cooked in water and sprinkle with lemon juice and herbs. Drink a glass of water **Calories:** 440
Midafternoon snack	Protein drink: Mix one serving protein powder with 4 oz water and 4 oz nonfat milk. Add one whole banana and blend. **Calories:** 240
Dinner	Chicken Meal: Prepare a skinless chicken breast by squeezing lemon juice over it. Grill until cooked. Serve with a portion of steamed brown rice and broccoli. **Calories:** 380
Late evening snack	One serving of low fat cereal or granola with 6 oz of skim milk. **Calories:** 250

Body Fat Blitz Sample Meal Plan

Breakfast	Egg white scramble: Mix five egg whites with one tbsp of nonfat milk. Cook in a nonstick pan coated with a non-fat cooking spray. Serve on one piece of whole-wheat toast. Drink one cup of black coffee or water. **Calories**: 230
Midmorning snack	Meal replacement: Mix one sachet of a meal-replacement powder with 12 oz cold water in a blender **Calories**: 340
Lunch	Tuna Meal: Drain one 6 oz can of water-packed tuna and squeeze some lemon juice over it. Serve with one portion (50g) of steamed rice. Drink a glass of ice water. **Calories**: 300
Midafternoon Snack	Protein drink: Mix one serving of protein powder with 4 oz water or 4 oz nonfat milk. Add one whole banana and blend. **Calories**: 240
Dinner	Chicken Meal: Prepare a skinless chicken breast by squeezing lemon juice over it. Grill until cooked. Serve with a 50 g portion of steamed brown rice and spinach or broccoli. **Calories**: 380
Late evening Snack	Eat half a low carb protein bar **Calories**: 150

Appendix 2

TRAINING, NUTRITION AND PROGRESS CHARTS

Use the following charts to plan and record your workouts, diet and progress.

Training Log

Date	Muscle	Exercise	Set 1 (Weight x Reps)	Set 2 (Weight x Reps)	Set 3 (Weight x Reps)

Note:

Workout time:

Personal Diet Chart

Meal	Time	Food	Calories	Protein	Carbs	Fat
1						
2						
3						
4						
5						
6						
Totals (Per day)						

Progress Chart

Measurements	Start	Month1	Month2	Month3	Month4	Month 5
Body Weight						
Body fat %						
Size: Waist Chest Arms Thighs						
Cardio time						
Strength (6 Reps) Bench Press Squat Bicep Curl						

Notes:

BIBLIOGRAPHY

Bone and Mineral Research, Wiley *online Library*, October 2017
Encyclopedia of Behavioral Medicine, *Marc D. Gellman & J. Rick Turner*, 2013
HHS physical activity guideline, KL Piercy · 2018
American Heart Association,
Obesity Journal, November 2017
Aging Clinical and Experimental Research, *Pedro Lopez, Ronei Silveira Pinto, Eduardo Lusa Cadore,* November 2017
AMA Psychiatry, Association of Efficacy of Resistance training with Depressive Symptoms: **Brett R. Gordon, MSc; Cillian P. McDowell, BSc; Mats Hallgren, PhD; et al.** une 2018.
Men's Body Sculpting, *Nick Evans*, 2014

www.ingramcontent.com/pod-product-compliance
Lightning Source LLC
LaVergne TN
LVHW010505160826
845677LV00012B/2658

* 9 7 9 8 8 4 6 6 1 1 1 0 8 *